Essentials of Enzymology

Essentials of Enzymology

Rufus O. Okotore

Copyright © 2015 by Rufus O. Okotore.

ISBN: Softcover   978-1-5035-2723-2
              eBook   978-1-5035-2722-5

All rights reserved. No part of this book may be reproduced or transmitted in any form or by any means, electronic or mechanical, including photocopying, recording, or by any information storage and retrieval system, without permission in writing from the copyright owner.

Any people depicted in stock imagery provided by Thinkstock are models, and such images are being used for illustrative purposes only.
Certain stock imagery © Thinkstock.

Print information available on the last page.

Rev. date: 03/10/2015

To order additional copies of this book, contact:
Xlibris
1-888-795-4274
www.Xlibris.com
Orders@Xlibris.com
696696

CONTENTS

Preface 11
Foreword 13

PART I: BASIC ENZYME CHEMISTRY AND PHYSIOLOGY

Chapter One: General Consideration On Enzymes 17
1.0   History of Enzymology..17
1.1   General Properties of Enzymes...20
1.2   Nomenclature And Classification 21
1.3   Summary...27

Chapter Two: Enzyme Physiology 29
2.0   Distribution of Enzymes 29
2.1   Extraction of Enzymes...36
2.2   Fractionation of Enzyme Preparation 36
2.3   Purification of Enzyme Preparation..39
2.4   Characterization of Enzyme Preparation 39

Chapter Three: Structure of Enzymes 41
3.0   Introduction..41
3.1   Classification And Structures of Amino Acids 42
3.2   Acid-Base Properties of Amino Acids 47
3.3   Structural Organisation of Enzymes 48
3.4   Coenzymes..55
3.5   Metalloenzymes 60

Chapter Four: Analytical Enzymology 63
4.0   Introduction..63
4.1   Measurement of Enzyme Levels..63
      4.1.1   Units of Measurement..64
4.2   Definitions of Enzyme Activity Parameters 65

4.3	Measurement of Catalytic Activity	66
4.4	Assay Techniques For Enzyme Activity	69
4.5	Factors Affecting Enzyme Activity	71

Review Questions 76
References 76

PART II: ENZYME KINETICS

Chapter Five: Enzyme Kinetics I 81
5.0 Introduction To Enzyme Kinetics 81
5.1 Order of Reactions 81
5.2 General Rate Equations For First Order Reactions 83
5.3 General Rate Equation For Second Order Reactions ... 84
5.4 Derivation of Michaelis-Menten Equation 86
5.5 Determination of The Kinetic Constants 89
5.7 Steady State Kinetics 94
5.8 Cases Where Intermediates Occuring After [ES] 96
5.9 Reversible Reaction 97
5.10 Measurement of Rate Constants 100
5.11 Rapid-Mixing And Quenching Techniques 101
5.12 Relaxation Methods 103

Chapter Six: Enzyme Kinetics II 105
6.0 Multisubstrate Enzyme Catalysed Reactions 105
6.1 Sequential Mechanism 106
6.2 Non-Sequential Mechanism (Ping-Pong) 107
6.3 Kinetics of Bisubstrate Reactions 108
6.4 Derivation of Rate Equation For Two-Substrate Reaction 109
6.5 Steady State Kinetics For Multi-Substrate Reactions ... 111
6.6 Non-Linear Kinetics 113
6.7 Ligand-Binding To Allosteric Protein 114
6.8 Kinetics of Ligand-Binding To Hemoproteins [Myoglobin & Haemoglobin] 116
6.9 Quantitative Analysis of Cooperativity 118
6.10 Kinetics of Ligand-Binding To An Allosteric Enzyme Molecule 119

Chapter Seven: Enzyme Kinetic III 122
7.0　Enzyme Inhibition...122
7.1　Types of Reversible Inhibition....................................125
7.2　Non-Competitive Inhibition.......................................128
7.3　Uncompetitive Inhibition 133
7.4　Mixed Inhibition 136
7.5　Determination of Inhibitor Constants 137
7.6　Summary 140
Review Questions 141
References..144

PART III: ENZYME CATALYSIS, MECHANISM AND REGULATION

Chapter Eight: Enzyme Catalysis And Mechanisms 149
8.0　Introduction..149
8.1　Acid-Base Catalysis 150
8.2　Nucleophilic And Electrophilic Catalysis
　　　[Covalent Catalysis]...152
8.3　Metal-Ion Catalysis 154
8.4　Enzyme Mechanisms 155
8.5　Chymotrypsin..156
8.6　Lysozyme 159

Chapter Nine: Active Site of Enzymes.. 162
9.0　General Consideration 162
9.1　Identification of Amino Acids At The Active Site
　　　of Enzymes...162
9.2　Substrate Labels 164
9.3　Pseudo-Substrate Labels 164
9.4　Affinity Labels 166
9.5　Cross-Linking Reagents...167

Chapter Ten: Regulation of Enzyme Activity 169
10.0　General Consideration 169
10.1　Types of Regulatory Mechanisms...............................171
10.2　Molecular Mechanisms of Allosteric Control............176
Review Questions 178
References..180

PART IV: APPLICATIONS OF ENZYMOLOGY

Chapter Eleven: Enzymes In Clinical Diagnosis 183
11.0   Introduction 183
11.1   Enzymes In Blood Plasma 183
11.2   Factors Which Control Enzyme Levels In Blood Plasma 185
11.3   Clinical Significance of Enzyme Analysis 187
11.4   Clinical Applications 189

Chapter Twelve: Enzyme Biotechnology 191
12.0   Introduction 191
12.1   Industrial Uses of Enzymes 192
12.2   Medicinal Applications of Enzymes 195
12.3   Immobilized Enzymes 198
12.4   Classification 199
12.5   Preparation of Immobilised Enzymes 200
12.6   Criteria For Choice of Carrier And Immobilization 201
12.7   Applications For Immobilized Enzymes 202
12.8   Enzyme Bioinformatics 202
Review Questions 204

Appendix 207
Glossary 215
Index 219

This book is dedicated to the memory of my late parents:
Pa Samuel Ogunjobi Okotore and Madam Abigail Keyede Okotore.
Also, it is affectionately dedicated to my wife and children.

PREFACE

Enzymology (the study of enzymes) is of special relevance and interest to both the biological and physical sciences.

Its practical applications in diverse human activities such as brewing; industrial fermentations, pest control, chemical and biological warfare to mention a few is not only well documented but equally well known.

This text has emerged from the synthesis of the lecture notes on enzymology courses for the undergraduate B.Sc (Hons) Biochemisty degree programme at the University of Lagos, Lagos Nigeria. It is a complete digest of the most important and relevant facts and information on the various topics in basic enzymology presented in a concise manner for easy assimilation. It is expected to augment the understanding of various specialised textbooks on Enzymology.

The book is in twelve chapters, which have been divided into four sections. Part 1 deals with the basic concepts in enzyme chemistry, while Part II is entirely devoted to Kinetics. The rigorous mathematical treatment of Enzyme Kinetics in many published works has been simplified and presented in a lucid comprehensible manner. Part III, deals with enzyme catalysis, mechanisms and regulation. Part IV which consists of two chapters discusses the application of enzymes in industry and medicine, enzyme biotechnology and bioinformatics.

The book is intended mainly for the undergraduate science students offering courses in enzymology, most especially those pursuing honours degree programme in Biochemistry and chemistry. It may also serve as a quick review text for the graduate students in the MSc degree programme in these disciplines.

Lastly, I wish to thank the various sets of B.Sc. (Hon.) biochemistry final year students and also the academic colleagues, for their criticisms. I thank Prof Adeyinka Afolayan, and Prof. Olorunsogo for reading through the manuscript and for the useful suggestions and advice towards the final preparation of the book.

I owe responsibility for other errors and omissions that may be quite apparent in the text. The reproductions of the diagrams, impressions from various sources are hereby acknowledged. I am grateful to the secretarial support from the teaching units, and the Dept. at various stages of preparation of the manuscript.

R.O. Okotore, PhD
Professor of Biochemistry

FOREWORD

In the last three decades, many specific text books or monographs on enzyme and protein science have appeared in the world market. More often, the emphasis in many of these monographs has been on the characteristics of purified enzymes without any in-depth reference about their importance to our everyday life. This book seeks to remedy that situation.

I am sure many senior undergraduate students, who consider their "enzymological pathway" difficult to tread on, will find the approach adopted by Prof. R.O. Okotore, an experienced teacher and investigator, who has taught and supervised many generations of students in this field, a soothing balm. There is also a lot to be gained by graduate students and even established investigators from the monograph. The style of writing is simple, lucid and personal. I therefore commend the book to all those who come across it.

ADEYINKA AFOLAYAN, Ph.D.
PROFESSOR OF BIOCHEMISTRY
DEPT OF BIOCHEMISTRY,
OBAFEMI AWOLOWO UNIVERSITY
ILE-IFE,
OSUN STATE
NIGERIA.

PART I

Basic Enzyme Chemistry And Physiology

CHAPTER ONE

General Consideration On Enzymes

1.0 HISTORY OF ENZYMOLOGY

The history of enzymology is comparatively recent. Although certain manifestations of the enzyme action, for example, fermentation, digestion and respiration had been known for a long time, the exact nature of the processes and the causing agents were unknown. Whilst, a few fundamental observations were made towards the beginning of the 19th century, the great developments in the field came during the last three or four decades of that century.

By 1920, there were only a dozen enzymes known; none had been isolated and also their nature was not clear. Presently, about 1000 different enzymes are known of which many have been partially purified and, in fact obtained pure and crystalline. The chemical structures of a considerable number have been well-established.

Historical Development

The first discovery of an enzyme was made by Payen and Persoz (1883) in Paris. They obtained from an aqueous extract of malt, by precipitation with alcohol; a substance, that could convert starch into sugar. Characteristically, this substance was inactivated by heating which is one of the characteristic properties of enzymes. The chemistry of the process was unknown and the factor was called "diastase" from the Greek word "for separation".

In 1836, Schawn extracted an active principle from the stomach wall of pigs which could digest food *in vitro*. This was called *pepsin*. In 1836, Berzelius put forward the concept of catalysis to explain the hastened hydrolysis of glucoside, amygdalin obtained from bitter almonds to yield benzylaldehyde, glucose and hydrogen cyanide by the active agent, emulsin.

The emulsin was present in the emulsion formed when the protein residue was extracted with water. Other examples of catalytic processes were the fermentation of sugar by yeast, the decomposition of hydrogen peroxide. However, the nomenclature of these new organic catalysts was confusing. Most scientists especially in France refer to these agents as "diastases".

Louis Pasteur (1822-1895) advanced that all the catalytic actions should be attributed to living organisms. He used the word 'ferment' to designate the entire group of catalysts. The word "ferment" was applied indiscriminately and no distinction between living organisms like yeast, and decay processes were made. This led to a good deal of confusion which at that time was generally referred to as "Liebig-Pasteur Controversy". The **reductionistic thesis** which regarded 'ferment' as being associated with decay and death, was proposed by Liebig in 1939.

Thus, decomposing ferments, were meant to depict the state of inner movements which act mechanically on other substances. On the other hand, Pasteur proposed that the action of fermentation was produced by living cells only. The proposed chemical reactions occurring in fermentations were considered as an essential part of life processes of the yeast. By mid-19th century, it was obvious that the digestive ferments were not microorganisms and that *ferment* consists of two separate entities, namely "organic ferments" which are yeast and micro-organisms and "inorganic ferments" that are enzymes.

Kühne (1878) introduced the name, **enzyme** ('in yeast') because these substances were inside the yeast and not the yeast itself. He emphasised that they could be found present in more complex organisms. This name has now been universally adopted. Buchner (1897) was able to extract from yeast, a cell-free juice which brings about the complete fermentation of sugar. This experiment opened a new field in enzyme chemistry. The possibility that a catalyst could be separated in solution from the cells which elaborated it led to the notion that other micro-organisms as well as plant and animal tissues could be subjected to the action of solvent to obtain enzymes.

Serious purification of enzymes did not start until the period (1922 - 1928), when Willstäther undertook the purification of "saccharase". In 1926, Sumner prepared the first crystalline enzyme, **urease,** from the jack-bean seeds. Northrop (1948) made classical isolation of several crystalline proteolytic enzymes.

The important enzymes known in the 19th century are listed in Table 1.1.

Table 1.1: Important enzymes discovered by 19th century

Name	Discovery	Isolation	Crystallisation
Diastase	Kirchhoff, (1814)	Payen and Persoz (1833)	Meyer *et al.* 1948
Pepsin	Eberle, 1934	Schwann, 1836	Northrop, 1930
Emulsin	Roubiquet, 1830	Liebig and Wohler (1837)	-
Invertase	Dubrunfaut, 1846	Berthelot, 1860	-
Urease	Fourcroy and Vanquelin 1799	Musculus, 1876	Sumner, 1926
Trypsin	Corvisart, 1857	Kuchnne, 1877	Northrop *et al.* 1931
Papain	Hughes, 1750	Wurtz *et al,* (1879)	Balls *et al.,* 1939

1.1 GENERAL PROPERTIES OF ENZYMES

Enzymes are organic molecules found in all living cells. They possess high molecular weights and are composed largely or entirely of protein. Like all catalysts, enzymes have the following properties:

(a) they act in extremely small quantities,
(b) they emerge unchanged intact from the reactions,
(c) they have no effect upon the final position of the equilibrium for the reaction; instead they merely accelerate its adjustments; and
(d) they lower the activation energy of the chemical reactions.

Apart from the aforementioned, they possess special unique features namely:

(i) They exhibit extremely high efficiency when compared to inorganic catalysts such as platinum and nickel.
(ii) The reactions which they catalyse proceed 10^8 to 10^{11} times faster than the non-enzymatic reactions under optimum conditions.
(iii) The number of substrate molecules metabolised per enzyme molecule (turnover number) is of magnitude 10^{10} to 10^{19}.
(iv) The reactions in which they are involved are very specific. This specificity is of four different types; absolute specificity; stereochemical specificity; reaction or linkage specificity and group specificity. For example, urease exhibits absolute specificity in action in that it catalyses the splitting of urea into ammonia and water only. D-amino acid oxidase exhibits stereochemical specificity in that it is specific for D-amino acids and will not affect the natural L-amino acids. The proteolytic enzymes exhibit group specificity, for they catalyse the hydrolysis of peptide bonds or of esters. These proteolytic enzymes: chymotrypsin, trypsin, thrombin vary in degree of substrate specificity. Thus, they also exhibit linkage specificity.
(v) The spectra of reactions often catalysed by enzymes are broad. These include, oxidation-reduction reactions, hydrolytic reactions, polymerisation, dehydration reactions,.
(vi) The enzyme activities are subject to a variety of controls, thus, highly regulated. Thus, the rate of synthesis, as well as their final concentration in the cell are under genetic control.

In some cases, enzymes are synthesised in an inactive form and then, activated at a physiologically appropriate time and place. Most proteolytic enzymes exist primarily as inactive forms called *zymogens;* and these undergo activation by cleavage of specific peptide bond to form the active forms. The mechanisms of the interconversion may be either through

(a) the activation of hydrolysis as exemplified by the zymogens, or
(b) through covalent modifications; that is the covalent insertion of a small group to the enzyme, such as the process observable in glycogen synthesis.

(vii) Enzymes are involved in the transformation of different kinds of energy. For example, the light energy is converted into chemical (bond) energy during photosynthesis and also the chemical energy can be converted to mechanical energy during muscle contraction. In all these cases, enzymes do play vital roles in the biochemical reactions.

1.2 NOMENCLATURE AND CLASSIFICATION

Enzymes were originally named according to their sources or according to the method of separation with which they were discovered. The prefix - "ase" was frequently added to the root of the name of the substrate, for example, urease catalyses the hydrolysis of urea; lipase is an enzyme that hydrolyses lipids. This system was applied to name types of enzymes such as proteases, oxidases and hydrolases. The discovery of so many enzymes and enzyme mechanisms in later years resulted in an unwieldy list of complex substrates and enzyme nomenclature. This situation prompted the need for a systematic arrangement and nomenclature so as to eliminate the inconsistencies in terminology. The task was assigned to a Commission on Enzymes of the International Union of Biochemistry.

1.2.1 Scheme of Classification and Numbering of Enzymes

The first Enzyme Commission, in its 1961 report, devised a system for classification of enzymes that also serves as a basis for assigning code numbers to them. These code numbers, prefixed by EC, which are now widely in use, contain four elements separated by points, with the following meaning:

(i) the first figure shows to which of the six main divisions (classes) the enzyme belongs,
(ii) the second figure indicates the sub-class,
(iii) the third figure gives the sub-sub-class,
(iv) the fourth figure is the serial number of the enzyme in its sub-sub-class.

The sub-classes and sub-sub-classes are formed according to principles as outlined in the most recent report of the Enzyme Commission (1978). The full key to the classification is given in the Appendix. Accordingly, the enzymes have been grouped into six major classes: oxidoreductases, transferases, hydrolases, lyases, isomerases and ligases, each having 4 to 13 subclasses.

1.2.2 Classification of Enzymes

(i) Oxido-Reductases

All enzymes which catalyze oxido-reduction reactions belong to this class. The substrate which is oxidised is regarded as the hydrogen donor. The systematic name is based on donor: acceptor oxidoreductase. The recommended name will be dehydrogenase but oxidase is only used in cases where O_2 is the acceptor.

The second figure in the code number of the oxidoreductases indicates the group in the hydrogen donor which undergoes oxidation:

1. denotes a CHOH-group,
2. an aldehyde - or keto-group, and so on, as listed in the Appendix.

The third figure, except in subgroups 1.11 and 1.15, indicates the type of acceptor involved:

1. denotes NAD(P),
2. a cytochrome,

3. molecular oxygen,
4. a disulphide,
5. a quinone or related compound etc.

It should be noted that in reactions with a nicotinamide coenzyme, this is always regarded as acceptor even if the direction of the reaction is not readily demonstrated. Although not used as a criterion of classification, the two hydrogen atoms at carbon-4 of the dihydropyridine ring of nicotinamide are located stereospecifically. The stereospecificity of a large number of dehydrogenases has been determined.

(ii) Transferases

Transferases are enzymes transferring a group, e.g. the methyl group or a glycosyl group, from one compound (generally regarded as a donor) to another compound (generally regarded as an acceptor). The systematic names are formed according to the scheme, donor: acceptor group transferase. The recommended names are normally formed according to acceptor group transferase or donor group transferase. In many cases, the donor is a cofactor (coenzyme) charged with the group to be transferred. A special case is that of the aminotransferases.

Some transferase reactions can be viewed in different ways. For example, the enzyme-catalysed reaction:

$$X - Y + Z = X + Z - Y \qquad (i)$$

may be regarded either as a transfer of the group Y from X to Z, or as a breaking of the X-Y bond by the introduction of Z. Where Z represents phosphate or arsenate, the process is often spoken of as 'phosphorolysis' or 'arsenolysis', respectively; and a number of enzyme names based on the pattern of phosphorylase action have come into use. These names are not suitable for a systematic nomenclature and it is better to regard them simply as Y-transferases.

Another problem is poised in the enzyme-catalysed transamination reactions.

$$R^1 - CHNH_2 - R^2 + R^3 - CO - R^4 \xrightarrow{Enzyme}$$
$$R^1 - CO - R^2 + R^3 - CHNH_2 - R^4 \qquad (2)$$

They involve the transfer of one electron pair and a proton, together with the *NH_2* group, from a primary amine to an "oxo" compound, according to the general equation [2].

The reaction can formally be considered as oxidative deamination of the donor (e.g. amino acid) linked with reductive amination of the acceptor (e.g. oxo acid), and the transaminating enzymes (pyridoxal-phosphate-proteins) might be classified as oxidoreductases.

However, the unique distinctive feature of the reaction is the transfer of the amino group (by a well-established mechanism involving covalent substrate-coenzyme intermediates), which justifies allocation of these enzymes among the transferases as a special subgroup 2.6.1, aminotransferases (Appendix).

(iii) Hydrolases

These enzymes catalyze the hydrolytic cleavage of C-O, C-N, C-C and some other bonds, including phosphoric anhydride bonds. Although, the systematic names always includes hydrolase, the recommended name is, in many cases, formed by the name of the substrate with the suffix "-ase".

A number of hydrolases acting on ester, glycosyl, peptide, amide or other bonds are known to catalyse not only hydrolytic removal of a particular group from their substrates, but likewise the transfer of this group to suitable acceptor molecules.

In principle, all hydrolytic enzymes might be classified as transferases, since hydrolysis itself can be regarded as transfer of a specific group to water as the acceptor. Yet, in most cases, the reaction with water as the acceptor was discovered earlier and is considered as the main physiological function of the enzyme. This is why such enzymes are classified as hydrolases rather than as transferases.

Some hydrolases (especially among the esterases and glycosidases) poise problems because they have a very wide specificity and it is not easy to decide if two preparations described by different authors (perhaps from different sources) have the same catalytic properties, or if they should be listed under separate entries. An example is vitamin A esterase (formerly EC 3.1.1.12, now believed to be identical with EC 3.1.1.1.).

Another problem is the so-called 'esterolytic' proteases, which hydrolyse ester bonds in appropriate substrates even more rapidly than natural peptide bonds. In this case, classification among the peptide hydrolases was based on historical priority and presumed physiological function.

The second figure in the code number of the hydrolases indicates the nature of the bond hydrolysed: 3.1 are the esterases, 3.2 the glycosidases, and so on (see Appendix I).

The third figure normally specifies the nature of the substrate e.g. in the esterases the carboxylic ester hydrolases (3.1.1), thiol ester hydrolases (3.1.2), phosphoric monoesterases (3.1.3); in the glycosidases, the O-glycosidases (3.2.1), N-glycosidases (3.2.2) etc. Exceptionally, in the case of the peptidyl-peptide hydrolases, the third figure is based on the catalytic mechanism as shown by active centre studies or the effect of pH.

(iv) Lyases

Lyases are enzymes cleaving C-C, C-N and other bonds by elimination leaving double bonds, or conversely adding groups to double bonds. The systematic name is formed according to the pattern: substrate group-lyases. The hyphen is an important part of the name, and to avoid confusion should not be omitted, e.g. hydro-lyase not 'hydrolyase'. In the recommended names, expressions like decarboxylase, aldolase, dehydratase (in case of elimination of water) are used. In case where the reverse reaction is much more important, or the only one demonstrated, synthase (not synthetase) may be used in the name. Various subclasses of the lyases include pyridoxal-phosphate enzymes that catalyse the elimination of β- or γ- substituent from an α- amino acid followed by a replacement of this substituent by some other group. In the overall replacement reaction, no unsaturated end-products is formed: therefore, these enzymes were formerly classified as alkyl-transferases (EC 2.5.1). However, there is ample evidence that the replacement is a two-step reaction involving the transient formation of enzyme bound, (or,) unsaturated amino acids. According to the rule, that the first reaction is indicative for classification, these enzymes are correctly classified as lyases. Examples are tryptophan synthase (EC 4.2.1.20) and cystathionine synthase (EC 4.2.1.22).

The second figure in the code number indicates the bond broken:

(a) 4.1 carbon-carbon-lyases,
(b) 4.2 carbon-oxygen-lyases and so on.

The third figure gives further information on the group eliminated (e.g. CO_2 in 4.1.1; H_2O in 4.2.1 (see Appendix).

(v) Isomerases

These enzymes catalyze geometric or structural changes within one molecule. According to the type of isomerism, they may be called racemases, epimerases, cis-trans-isomerases, tautomerases, mutases or cyclo-isomerases. In some cases, the interconversion in the substrate is brought about by an intra-molecular oxidoreduction (5.3); (see Appendix). Since the hydrogen donor and acceptor are the same molecule, and no oxidised product appears, they are not classified as oxidoreductases, even if they may contain firmly bound NAD (P)+.

The subclasses are formed according to the type of isomerism, the sub-subclasses are formed according to the type of substrates (see Appendix).

(vi) Ligases (Synthetases)

Ligases are enzymes catalyzing the joining together of two molecules coupled with the hydrolysis of a pyrophosphate bond in ATP or a similar triphosphate. The bonds formed are often high energy bonds. The systematic names are formed on the system, X:Y ligase (ADP-forming). In the recommended nomenclature, the synthetase may be used, if no other short term (e.g. carboxylase) is available (see Appendix).

1.3 SUMMARY

The Six Major Classes of Enzymes

1. *Oxidoreductases:* These enzymes are involved in the catalysis of the oxidation - reduction reactions in the living cell.
2. *Transferases:* These enzymes catalyze the transfer of a chemical group from one substrate to another. Thus, they are involved in group transfer reactions. These groups include amino, methyl, alkyl, acyl and those containing phosphorus or sulphur.
3. *Hydrolases:* Enzymes in this group catalyze hydrolytic reactions and include digestive enzymes such as amylases, proteases and lipases.
4. *Lyases:* These enzymes catalyze the addition of groups to double bonds and vice-versa. They are involved in the removal of chemical groups without hydrolysis. They act on C=O, C=N and C=C bonds.
5. *Isomerases:* This group of enzymes catalyzes isomerisation reactions.
6. *Ligases* (Synthetases). These enzymes catalyze the condensation of two molecules with the breaking of a pyrophosphate bond of ATP or similar nucleoside triphosphate.

Many trivial names are in frequent use. These names ending with 'ase' give information concerning the nature of the substrate involved and the nature of the catalyzed reaction. Few examples are illustrated as follows:

(i) Dehydrogenases: These are enzymes which catalyze dehydrogenation of their substrates with a molecule other than molecular oxygen as hydrogen acceptor.
(ii) Oxidases: These enzymes catalyze oxidation of their substrates, with molecular oxygen as the electron acceptor.

(iii) Kinases: These enzymes catalyze the transfer of phosphate from ATP or from another nucleoside triphosphate to their substrates.
(iv) Phosphatases: This class of enzymes catalyze the hydrolytic cleavage of phosphate esters.
(v) Phosphorylases: These are enzymes that catalyze the addition of the elements of phosphoric acid across glycosyl or related linkages.
(vi) Mutases: They catalyze the migration of a phosphate group from one hydroxyl group to another within the same molecule.

CHAPTER TWO

Enzyme Physiology

2.0 DISTRIBUTION OF ENZYMES

Enzymes are mostly contained in cells and component parts. The cell nucleus is rich in enzymes for the metabolism of nucleic acids and for protein synthesis. The cytoplasm contains enzymes that participate in glycolysis, transaminations, the metabolism of galactose, fructose, and the synthesis of urea. The cell membrane is rich in adenosine triphosphatase. The endoplasmic structure, likewise, are rich in enzymes; so also the mitochondria, the endoplasmic reticulum, lysosomes and other sub-cellular structures. [Tables 2.2 - 2.6]. These structures can be isolated from the disrupted cells by fractionation procedure and differential centrifugation, see Scheme 1. The marker enzymes to ascertain the purity of the respective subcellular fractions are stated in Table 2.1.

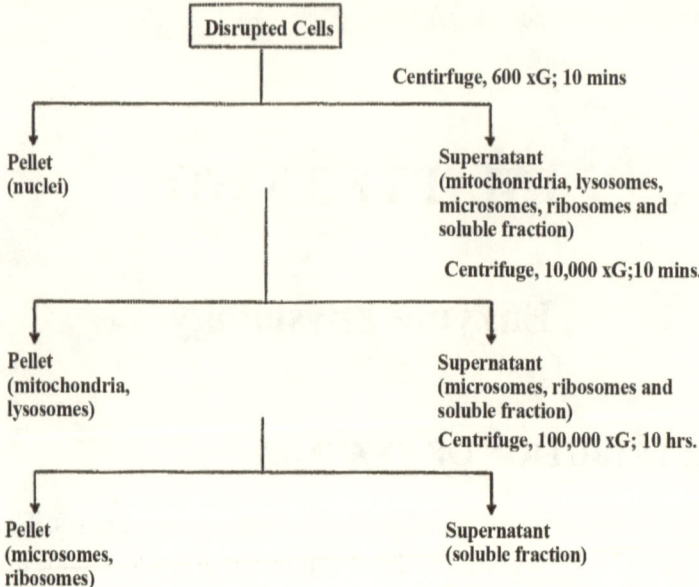

Scheme I: Procedure for subcellular fractionation by differential centrifugation

Enzyme systems exhibit regular formations especially within the cell, where the formations represent metabolic segments. Furthermore, the enzyme formation within an entire origin is also of prime importance; - for example, the enzymes within the liver cells show different levels of activity in different parts of the hepatic lobule. With regard to the strength of their binding, the intracellular enzymes may be classified into (i) lyoenzymes, which are easily extractable; (ii) endoenzymes, which are extractable only after destruction of cell membrane; and (iii) desmoenzymes, which are firmly bound to mitochondria or nuclei and capable of release only after vigorous intervention. This classification possesses practical relevance concerning the rate of release of individual enzymes from cells into the blood in pathological conditions.

Table 2.1: Marker enzymes used in subcellular fractionation

Marker Enzyme	Subcellular Fraction
DNA nucleotidyl transferase	Nuclei
NMN adenyl transferase	Nuclei
Succinate dehydrogenase	Mitochondria
Cytochrome- 6- oxidase	Mitochondria
Glucose 6-phosphatase	endoplasmic reticulum
Acid phosphatase	Lysosomes
Ribonuclease	Lysosomes
Catalase	Peroxisomes
Urate oxidase	Peroxisomes
5-Nucleotidase	plasma membrane
Glucose 6-phosphate dehydrogenase	Cytosol
Lactate dehydrogenase	Cytosol
6-Phosphofructokinase	Cytosol

Table 2.2: Enzymes present in the nucleus

1. Enzymes in the soluble space
    Glycolytic enzymes
    Pentose phosphate pathway enzymes
    Lactate dehydrogenase
    Malate dehydrogenase
    Isocitrate dehydrogenase
    Arginase
2. Enzymes bound to chromatin
    RNA nucleotidyl transferase II
    RNA nucleotidyl transferase III
    Nucleoside triphosphatase
    DNA nucleotidyl transferase
    NMN adenyl transferase

3. Enzymes concentrated in the nucleolus
   RNA nucleotidyl transferase I
   RNA methyl transferases
   Ribonuclease
4. Enzymes bound to membranes
   Glucose 6-phosphatase
   Acid phosphatase

Table 2.3: Principal enzymes or groups of enzymes present in the mitochondrion

1. Matrix
   Tricarboxylic acid cycle enzymes except succinate dehydrogenase
   Enzymes catalysing P-oxidation of fatty acids
   Pyruvate carboxylase
   Phosphoenolpyruvate carboxykinase (Pigeon liver)
   Carbamoyl-phosphate synthetase
   Ornithine carbamoyl transferase Glutamate dehydrogenase
2. Inner membrane
   Succinate dehydrogenase (NADH dehydrogenase) + associated respiratory chain
   Adenosine triphosphatase
   3-Hyroxybutyrate dehydrogenase
   Carnitine palmitoyl transferase
   Glycerol 3-phosphate dehydrogenase (FAD enzyme)
   a-Aminolevulinate synthase
   Hexokinase
   Cytochrome c oxidase
3. Intermembrane space
   Adenylate kinase
   Nucleoside diphosphate kinase
   Nucleoside monophosphate kinase
   L-xylulose-reductase

4. Outer membrane
   NADH dehydrogenase (rotenone insensitive)
   Cytochrome b_5 reductase
   Amine oxidase (flavin-containing)
   Kynureninase
   Acyl-CoA synthetase
   Glycerophosphate acyl transferase
   Choline phospho transferase
   Adenylate kinase
   Hexokinase
   Phospholipase A_2

Table 2.4: Enzymes present in lysosomes

1. Proteolytic enzymes
   Cathepsins B, D, G, L
   Elastase
   Collagenase
2. Hydrolysis of glycosides
   β-D-glucuronidase
   β-N-acetyl-D-hexosaminidase
   Lysozyme
   Neuraminidase
3. Hydrolysis of nucleic acids
   Deoxyribonuclease II
   Ribonuclease II
4. Hydrolysis of lipids
   Phospholipases A, and A_2
   Cholesterol esterase
5. Others
   Acid phosphatase
   Aryl sulphatase

Table 2.5: Principal enzymes of the endoplasmic reticulum

Enzyme or group of enzymes	Location
Cholesterol biosynthetic enzymes	* smooth endoplasmic reticulum
Steroid hydroxylation enzymes	smooth endoplasmic reticulum
Carnitine acyl transferase Fatty acid elongating enzymes (C_{16} - C_{24})	
Glycerolphosphate acyl transferase	smooth endoplasmic reticulum
D_{ring}-metabolising enzymes (aromatic ring hydroxylation, side chain oxidation, deamination, dealkylation, dehalogenation)	
Protein synthesis	* rough endoplasmic reticulum,
Glucose 6-phosphatase, Adenosine triphosphatase	cytoplasmic side of rough endoplasmic reticulum,
Cytochrome b_5 reductase	luminal side of rough endoplamic reticulum.
NADPH-cytochrome reductase	cytoplasmic side of rough endoplasmic reticulum
GDP mannose &-D-mannosyltransferase	cytoplasmic side of rough endoplasmic reticulum
Nucleoside diphosphatase	luminal side of endoplasmic reticulum
D-glucoronidase	luminal side of rough endoplasmic reticulum
UDP glucuronosyltransferase 5'Nucleotidase	cytoplasmic side of rough endoplasmic reticulum
Cholesterol acyltransferase	cytoplasmic side of rough endoplasmic reticulum

Table 2.6: Enzymes or groups of enzymes present in the cytosol

1. Carbohydrate metabolism
   Glycolytic enzymes including phosphorylase, phosphorylase kinase and protein kinase
   Glycogen synthase
   Fructose-bisphosphatase
   Phosphoenolpyruvate carboxykinase (rat liver)
   Enzymes of the pentose phosphate pathway
   Malate dehydrogenase
   Isocitrate dehydrogenase
   Lactate dehydrogenase
   Citrate (Pro-3S)-lyase
   Malate dehydrogenase (oxaloacetate-decarboxylating (NADP+))
   Giucose-l-phosphate uridylyltransferase
2. Lipid metabolism
   Acetyl-CoA carboxylase
   Fatty acid synthetase complex
   Glycerol-3-phosphate dehydrogenase (NAD+)
3. Amino acid and protein metabolism
   Aspartate aminotransferase
   Alanine aminotransferase
   Arginase
   Argininosuccinate lyase
   Aminoacyl-t RNA synthetases
4. Nucleic acid synthesis
   Nucleoside kinase
   Nucleotide kinase

2.1 EXTRACTION OF ENZYMES

The organelle is first isolated as the first step and the cells are then disrupted. The simplest method is to grind the tissue with a pestle in a mortar, sometimes with the addition of washed white sand or any other abrasive materials. Alternatively, the tissue can be forced in a press, through minute holes causing disintegration of the cells. More sophisticated methods include bursting the cells by osmotic shock and submitting them to ultrasonic vibrations. Homogenisers which are used in households have also been employed to achieve a shearing effect rather than crushing force thus minimising damage. In this case, the tissue is cut into small pieces in water or buffer, then as the sharp blade rotate at high speed, not only cutting the tissue but causing cavitation which helps to sheer the cells into smaller fragments. Once the cell membranes are ruptured, all kinds of abnormal enzymatic reactions can occur, so these reactions have to be inhibited so as to avoid chemical damage to the enzyme preparation. Two general procedures that have been found useful involve rapid breaking process and operating at very low temperatures.

The various procedures for the preparation of homogenates and the disintegration of cells are outlined in Table 2.7. As aforementioned, the most abundant source of an enzyme is frequently within a particulate. The fractionating techniques for obtaining the fractions of interest are stated in Table 2.8.

2.2 FRACTIONATION OF ENZYME PREPARATION

The disruption of cells leads to freeing of enzymes in solution. Debris of tissue fibres and other contaminants need to be removed, so various fractionating procedures are often carried out. These include fractional precipitation by change of pH; fractional denaturation by heating; fractional precipitation with organic solvents such as butanol, acetone; fractional precipitation by salts such as ammonium sulphate, sodium sulphate, or fractional adsorption on some materials such as charcoal, earth, celite. Of all, the salt precipitation with ammonium sulphate has been widely employed. Frequently, a combination of procedures are utilised to obtain product free from contaminants. A greater degree of purity is achieved through column chromatography on cellulose ion-exchangers: CM-cellulose, DEAE-cellulose. Recently, matrices which combine molecular sieve and ion-exchange properties have been introduced, for example, SE-Sephadex and DEAE-Sephadex beads. SE-Sephadex and DEAE-Sephadex beads are available from many commercial houses.

Table 2.7: Methods for the preparation of homogenates and for the disintegration of cells

Type of homogenate	Method	Tissue
(a) Wet homogenate	(I) Mechanical homogenisation	
	(a) Grinding with sand, aluminium powder, glass powder, diatomaceous earth.	Muscle, Bacteria
	(b) Pestle homogeniser	Muscle
	(c) Glass-bead homogeniser	Bacteria, Yeast
	(d) Blade homogeniser	Muscle
	(II) Sonic homogenisation	
	Ultrasonic homogeniser	bacteria, yeast
	(III) Thermal disintegration	Universal
	Freezing and thawing	Application
	Freezing with liquid N_2, liquid air	
	(IV) Chemical disintegration	
	isopentanol, butanol, digitonin, petroleum-ether	erythrocytes, mitochondria, muscle

	(v) Biological-enzymatic disintegration	
	autolysis, maceration, use of lysozyme and bacterial proteases	yeast, lysozyme, bacteria, muscle.
(b) Dry homogenate	homogenisation by dehydration; icetone; lyophilisation	universal dehydration application

Table 2.8: Methods for Tissue and Cell fractionation

Fraction	Method	Mode of Instrument Operation
Homogeneous cell suspension	Differential centrifugation and differential partition	Centrifuge up to 8,000 x G
Cell-free supernatant	Homogenisation; centrifugation	Centrifuge up to 10,000 x G
Cell nuclei	Homogenisation; differential centrifugation	Centrifuge up to 11,000 x G
Mitochondria sarcosomes	Homogenisation; differential centrifugation	Centrifuge up to 15,000 x G.
Sub-mitochondrial particles	Homogenisation, (sonic, chemical)	Ultracentrifuge up to 10,000 x G.
Microsomes	Differential centrifugation	Ultracentrifuge up to 100,000 x G
Ribosomes	As above for microsomes	Ultracentrifuge 13,000 to 198,000 x G
Particle-free	Centrifugation after separation of microsomes	Ultracentrifuge above 100,000 x G.

2.3 PURIFICATION OF ENZYME PREPARATION

Invariably, fairly pure enzyme preparation is obtained after the column chromatography on any of the aforementioned resins. The extent of purity can be ascertained by electrophoretic techniques or ultracentrifugation approach. In either case, a single band if observable indicates an homogeneous preparation.

However, if there are still contaminating species; such a preparation can be subjected to any of the following chromatographic techniques; namely ion-exchange; sephadex, (DEAE-Sephadex, SE-Sephadex) or affinity chromatography. An excellent treatise on the principles, operation and application of these techniques have been documented by a commercial firm, ***Pharmacia Fine Chemicals***; Sweden.

Criteria for Purity

An enzyme preparation is considered pure, if it fulfills at least two of the following criteria, namely:

(a) exhibits a single band on electrophoresis in charged polyacrylamide gels;
(b) single band on uncharged gels that contain denaturing agent, sodium dodecyl sulphate (SDS);
(c) exhibits a symmetrical distribution pattern from ultracentrifugation data;
(d) elutes as a single component in either ion-exchange or gel-filtration chromatography.

2.4 CHARACTERIZATION OF ENZYME PREPARATION

The final stage in the isolation and identification of a pure homogeneous enzyme preparation involves the characterization procedure. The characteristics entail the following parameters:

(a) the determination of the size or molecular size of the enzyme. This can be carried out by the gel-filtration approach using in conjunction some standard proteins of known molecular weights, the amino acid compositional data,

(b) determination of the binding constant (Michaeli's constant, K_m),
(c) the determination of pH optimum, and optimum temperature,
(d) the effect of activators and inhibitors on enzyme activity.
(e) Analysis of the 3-D, the three dimensional topography, hence the structure, by the X-ray diffraction technique is attempted.

CHAPTER THREE

Structure Of Enzymes

3.0 INTRODUCTION

Enzymes are protein molecules. These are macromolecules with molecular weights range 10,000 to 10^6. They consist of large number of amino acids units or residues covalently linked together to form unbranched chains. The monomer units (amino acids) are in a defined order. There are twenty amino acids commonly encountered in the enzyme (protein) molecule. The general formula of a naturally occurring amino acid may be represented as:

$$R - \underset{\underset{NH_2}{|}}{\overset{\overset{H}{|}}{C}} - COOH$$

(R = side chain)

The amino group is on the carbon atom adjacent to the carboxyl group; so the amino acids having this general formula are known as alpha (α) amino acid. The naturally occurring amino acids found in proteins have the L-configuration with respect to the reference standard, D-glyceraldehyde.

3.1 CLASSIFICATION AND STRUCTURES OF AMINO ACIDS

The amino acids in enzyme proteins may be classified according to the chemical nature (aliphatic, aromatic and basic) of their R groups (Table 3) or on the polarity of the R group or residue. The latter emphasises the functional role these amino acids play in the proteins. Accordingly, there are four major divisions (Table 3.2):

1. non-polar or hydrophobic;
2. polar but uncharged;
3. polar with negative charge at physiological pH, and
4. polar with a positive charge at physiological pH.

1. Amino Acids with Non-polar Or Hydrophobic R Groups

In this group are amino acids with aliphatic residues, viz: alanine, valine, isoleucine, leucine, methionine and also aromatic residues; phenylalanine and tryptophan. In addition, there is proline, whose nitrogen atom is present as a secondary amine rather than a primary amine.

$$H_3C-\underset{NH_2}{\overset{H}{\underset{|}{C}}}-CO_2H$$

L-Alanine

$$\underset{CH_3}{\overset{CH_3}{\diagdown}}CH-\underset{NH_2}{\overset{H}{\underset{|}{C}}}-COOH$$

L-Valine

$$\underset{CH_3}{\overset{CH_3}{\diagdown}}CH-CH_2-\underset{NH_2}{\overset{H}{\underset{|}{C}}}-COOH$$

L-Leucine

$$\text{C}_6\text{H}_5-CH_2-\underset{NH_2}{\overset{H}{\underset{|}{C}}}-COOH$$

L-Phenyl alanine

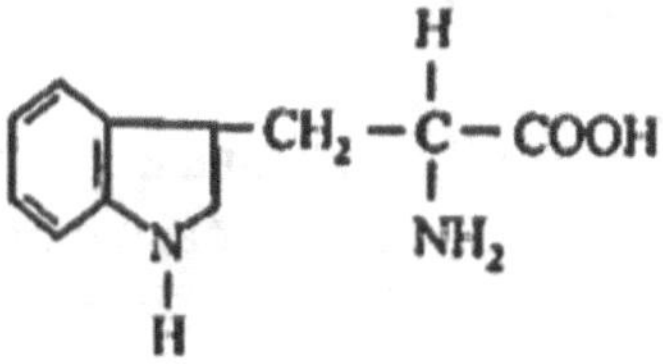

L-Trytophan

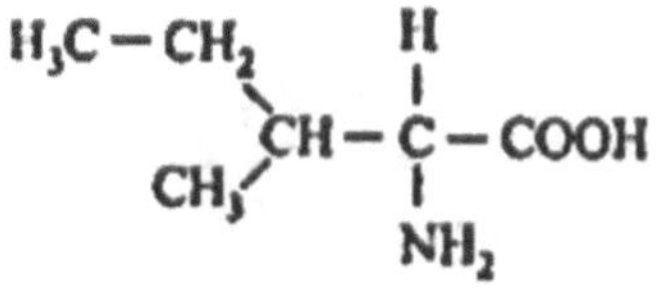

L-Isoleucine

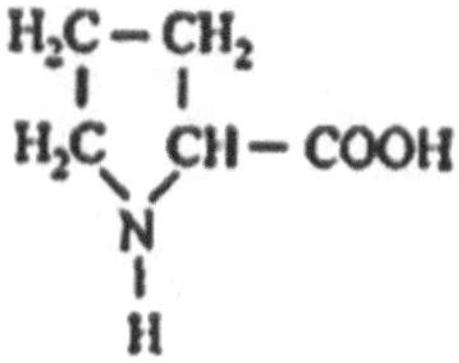

L-Proline

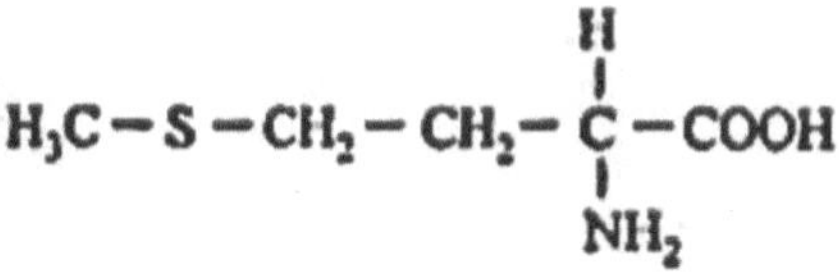

L-Methionine

2. Amino Acids with Polar But Uncharged R Groups

The amino acids in this group contain polar R residues which participate in hydrogen bond formation. Some possess a hydroxyl group (serine, threonine and tyrosine) or sulfhydryl group (cysteine) or amide groups (asparagine and glutamine). Glycine which has 'H' as the R group is included in this group.

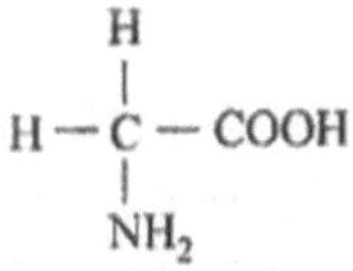

L-Glycine

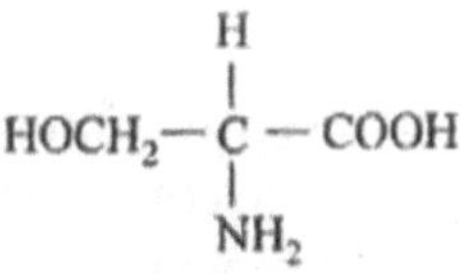

L-Serine

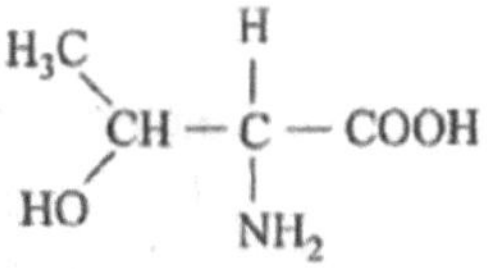

L-Threonine

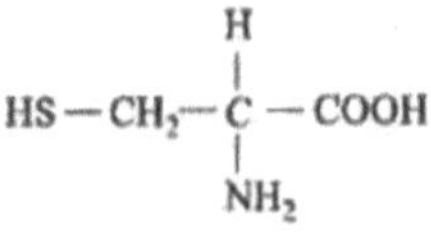

L-Cysteine

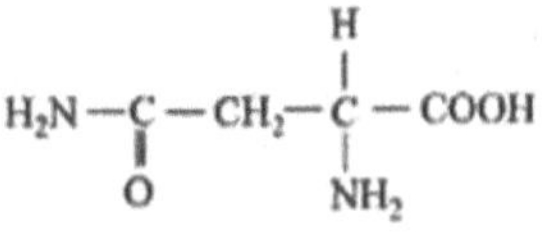

L-Asparagine

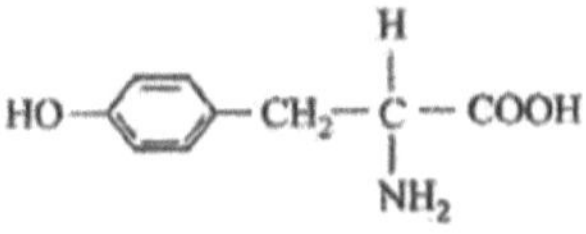

L-Tryosine

3. Amino Acids with Positively Charged "R Groups"

There are three amino acids, namely histidine, lysine and arginine in this group. Histidine has a weakly basic (pK = 6.0) imidazole group. It has a proton that dissociates in the neutral pH range, hence, this property plays significant role in the catalytic function of enzymes where any histidine residue is involved in the active site. Arginine contains a strong basic guanidinium group (pK=12.5); whilst lysine has second (epsilon, ε) amino group (pK=10.5).

$$H_2N-CH_2-CH_2-CH_2-CH_2-\underset{NH_2}{\overset{H}{\underset{|}{\overset{|}{C}}}}-COOH$$

L-Lysine

$$H_2N-\underset{NH}{\overset{}{\underset{\|}{C}}}-NH-CH_2-CH_2-CH_2-\underset{NH_2}{\overset{H}{\underset{|}{\overset{|}{C}}}}-COOH$$

L-Arginine

4. Amino Acids with Negatively Charged "R Group"

This group includes the two dicarboxylic amino acids - aspartic acid and glutamic acid. At neutral pH, the second carboxyl group has pKa_2 of 3.9 and 4.3 respectively. These dissociate giving a net charge of -1 to these compounds.

$$HOOC-CH_2-CH_2-\underset{NH_2}{\overset{H}{\underset{|}{\overset{|}{C}}}}-COOH \qquad HOOC-CH_2-\underset{NH_2}{\overset{H}{\underset{|}{\overset{|}{C}}}}-COOH$$

L-Glutamic acid   L-Aspartic acid

Table 3.1: Classification of Amino Acids in Enzyme Protein Based on Chemical Nature of R Group

		R group
I.	Aliphatic amino acids	
	Glycine (gly)	-H
	Alanine (ala)	$-CH_3$
	Valine (val)	$-CH(CH_3)_2$
	Leucine (leu)	$-CH_2.CH(CH_3)_2$
	Isoleucine (ile)	$-CH(CH_3)CH_2.CH_3$
II.	Acidic amino acids	
	Aspartic acid (asp)	$-CH_2.CO_2H$
	Glutamic acid (glu)	$-CH_2.CH_2.CO_2H$
III.	Acid amides	
	Asparagine (asn)	$-CH_2.CO.NH_2$
	Glutamine (gln)	$-CH_2.CH_2.CO.NH_2$
IV.	Basic amino acids	
	Lysine (lys)	$-(CH_2)_4NH_2$
	Histidine (his)	(imidazole ring: N=, NH)
	Arginine (arg)	$-(CH_2)_3.NH.C(:NH)NH_2$
V.	Hydroxy amino acids	
	Serine (ser)	$-CH_2.OH$
	Threonine (thr)	$-CH(OH).CH_3$
VI.	Sulphur-containing amino acids	
	Cysteine (cysH)	$-CH_2.SH$
	Cystine (cys)	$-CH_2.S.S.CH_2-$
	Methionine (met)	$-(CH_2)_2.S.CH_3$
VII.	Aromatic amino acids	
	Phenylalanine (phe)	$-CH_2-$(phenyl ring)

Tyrosine (tyr) $-CH_2-\langle\rangle-OH$

Tryptophan (try) (—CH₂— attached to indole ring with NH)

VIII. Imino acid
Proline (pro) (pyrrolidine ring: H₂C—CH₂, H₂C, HC—COOH, N—H)

Structurally, the simplest amino acid is glycine which contains a hydrogen atom as its side chain. Alanine has a methyl group as its side chain. Those which contain hydrocarbon side chains include valine, leucine, isoleucine and proline. However, proline differs from all the other amino acids in containing a secondary amine rather than a primary amine. (Table 3.1). It is generally referred to as an imino acid rather than amino acid. The side chain of proline is bounded to both the amino group and the α-carbon, thereby forming a cyclic structure.

Two amino acids, serine and threonine contain an aliphatic hydroxyl group. There are three common aromatic amino acids: phenylalanine, tyrosine and tryptophan. At physiological pH, all the side chains of the amino acids stated so far are uncharged. However, at this neutral pH, lysine and histidine may be positively charged or neutral depending on its local environment. The negatively charged side chains are those of glutamic acid and aspartic acid. Thus, these amino acids are called glutamate and aspartate, whereas the uncharged derivatives, are glutamine and asparagine respectively, which contain a terminal amide group rather than a carboxylate.

The remaining amino acids in the basic set of twenty found in proteins are cysteine and methionine, whose side chains contain a sulphur atom.

Table 3.2: Classification of Amino Acids
Based on the Polarity of R Group

GROUP I			GROUP II		
Non-Polar			Neutral-Polar		
Amino Acid	3-LS	1-LS	Amino Acid	3-LS	1-LS
Alanine	Ala	A	Serine	Ser	S
Valine	Val	V	Threonine	Thr	T
Isoleucine	lie	I	Cysteine	Cys	C
Leucine	Leu	L	Tyrosine	Tyr	Y
Proline	Pro	P	Glycine	Gly	G
Phenylalanine	Phe	F	Asparagine	Asp	N
Tryptophan	Trp	W	Glutamine	Gin	Q
Methionine	Met	M			

GROUP III			GROUP IV		
Positively-charged R group			Negatively-charged R group		
Amino Acid	3-LS	1-LS	Amino Acid	3-LS	1-LS
Lysine	Lys	K	Aspartic Acid	Asp	D
Histidine	His	H	Glutamic Acid	Glu	E
Arginine	Arg	R	Asparagine/ Aspartic Acid	Asx	B
			Glutamine/ Glutamic Acid	Glx	Z

Note: LS - Letter Symbol

3.2 ACID-BASE PROPERTIES OF AMINO ACIDS

(a) The acid-base properties of amino acids are due to the presence of at least an amino group and a carboxyl group in each molecule.
(b) In proteins, all except the terminal ;-amino and ;-carboxyl functions are masked; so the ionisable groups on the side chains of amino acids largely determine the acid-base properties (Table 3.2).

(c) The acid-base groups provide the basis for several important biochemical separation methods, for example, electrophoresis, thin-layer chromatography and ion-exchange chromatography.

(d) According to the Browstead-Lowry definitions of an acid (i.e. proton donor) and a base (a proton acceptor), all the functional groups in the enzyme molecule exhibit acid-base properties. Hence,

(i) An amino acid possesses at least two ionizable groups since they have two acid dissociation constants within the pH range 1-13 (one of $pK_a = 3$ and the second, near $pK_a = 10$). The pK_a values of the characteristic side chains of amino acids are presented in Table 3.3.

(ii) An amino acid exists in water entirely in the dipolar form at neutral pH ($pK_a = 7.0$). So, it is rather soluble in water, but it is less soluble in non-polar solutions. It also has large dipole moments.

(iii) Amino acids possess isoelectric points whose values are equal to half the sum total of dissociation constants (pK_a) of the acidic and basic groups in the molecule, that is,

$$pI = \frac{1}{2}(pK_a + pK_b)$$

3.3 STRUCTURAL ORGANISATION OF ENZYMES

Generally, the enzyme protein molecule is organised into four structural levels called primary, secondary, tertiary and quaternary:

(i) Primary Structure

The primary structure refers to the sequence, number and type of amino acid residues in the enzyme molecule. The sequence refers to the way in which amino acids are arranged in the molecule. The primary structure is stabilised by the peptide bonds between the amino acids and also the covalent disulfide linkages between the polypeptide chains.

(ii) Secondary Structure

The secondary structure is one which is due to the formation of hydrogen bonds between the component of the linkages itself.

From studies of the x-ray diffraction of crystalline low-molecular weight amides, Pauly & Corey proposed a set of standard experimental data which could lead to achieving a stable secondary structures, thus:

(a) peptide group must be planar and bond angles and lengths identified to those found in crystals of simple amides.
(b) every carboxyl oxygen and amide nitrogen must be involved in hydrogen bond formation.
(c) hydrogen-bonded hydrogens lie close to a line joining the oxygen and nitrogen atoms involved in the formation of the bond.
(d) the operation in going from one residue to the next (in terms for example, of translation along or rotation around a central axis) be the same for every residue.

So, the acceptable structures that meet these requirements fall into two general categories:

(a) helical structures derived from formation of intramolecular hydrogen bonds, and
(b) sheet structures derived from formation of intermolecular hydrogen bonds. Among the many possible helical structures considered by Pauling, Corey and other workers, only one fully meets all the specifications for maximum stability. This is termed the α-helix. This α-helix is characterised by a translation along a central axis parallel to the long axis of the axis of 5.4 A per turn. A complete turn is made for every 3.6 residues (Figure 3.3). Thus, the translation per residue is 1.5A, and the rotation per residue is **100°**.

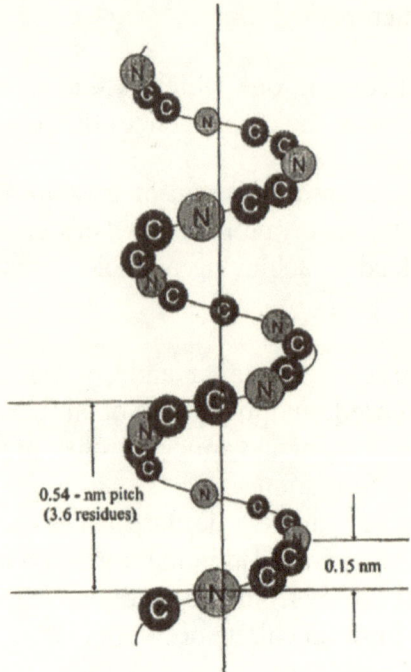

Figure 3.3: Orientation of the main chain atoms of a peptide about the axis of an α-helix

The side-chains of the amino acid residues bristle out from the helix. Each carboxyl oxygen and amide nitrogen is involved in hydrogen bond formation; carboxyl oxygens are hydrogen-bonded to amide nitrogens three residues back in the peptide chain. Thus, the repeating hydrogen-bonded unit may be visualised as follows:

$$-\overset{H}{\underset{|}{N}}-(-CHR-\overset{O}{\underset{\|}{C}}-\overset{H}{\underset{|}{N}}-)-C_\alpha$$

Proteins that contain helical structure may either be globular or fibrous. The sheet structures that result from formation of intermolecular hydrogen bonds are of two principal types, both consistent with the requirements of Pauling, Corey and Branson. These are termed the parallel and anti-parallel sheets. The contrast to the; α-helix, the hydrogen bonds in the sheet structures are oriented nearly perpendicularly to the long axis of the polypeptide chain. Proteins that contain sheet structures are fibrous and are generally insoluble in aqueous solvents.

(iii) The Tertiary Structure is the overall three-dimensional shape of a protein. It is stabilised partly by hydrogen bonds and partly by many weak interactions between side-chains which are widely separated from each other in the linear sequence of amino acids. These forces include electrostatic interactions, hydrophobic interactions and dipole-dipole moments. The term, conformation is often used to cover both the secondary and the tertiary structure of a protein.

(iv) The Quaternary Structure, which is the fourth level of organisation, is applicable to any protein in which the native molecule is composed of several separate sub-units. It refers to the way in which these units are grouped together.

3.3.1 X-Ray crystallography of Enzyme molecule

This is a physical analytical technique that involved the application of X-ray diffraction method. X-rays are electromagnetic radiations of wavelength, dimension, 0.1nm to 1.0nm (1-10Å) which is comparable to the intermolecular spacings in a crystal. Crystals are comprised of orderly arrangement of molecules, which form crystal lattices or space lattices. The lattices acts as a three-dimensional diffraction grating towards a monochromatic beam of X-rays. When the X-rays beams bombard the crystals, they are partly reflected, partly transmitted through and also scattered by the atoms in the crystal molecule as a number of diffracted ray beams. If a photographic plate is placed behind the crystal, these diffracted rays make their appearances on the plate as spots which represent the diffraction phenomenon at various planes. The complete array of spots is called the *diffraction pattern*. **From the consideration of the intensity of the spots in the pattern, and the distribution of electron density in the crystal, if when subjected to Fourier mathematical transforms, can assist to obtain an image of the protein molecule. This solution is possible only when the phases of the diffracted rays are known. This problem is solved by diffusing heavy metal atoms, such** as uranium, lead, mercury into specific sites in the crystal, but without distorting the crystal lattices. The metal ions often scatter the X-rays more strongly than the atoms of the protein molecule. Thus, by measuring the differences in electron density maps obtained from the data for the enzyme protein crystal in the presence of metal ions and that without the metal ions, the actual phases of the diffracted rays can be obtained. The Fourier transforms aid to generate the electron density maps which are then used to construct computer-generated three-dimensional models. The accuracy with which these can be made depends on the resolution of the X-ray diffraction method. The structural features which are observable at specific resolution range are stated below (Table 3.3).

Table 3.3: Resolution and structural information

Resolution 1 Å = 0.1 nm	Structural features observable
5.5	(i) Overall shape of molecule visible (ii) Helical conformations are seen as rods of strong intensity.
3.5	The main chains (polypeptide) are visible but usually with some ambiguities
3.0	The side chains (amino acids) are partially resolved.
2.5	The side chains (amino acids) are well-resolved; so also the plane of the peptide bond. Atoms can be located to about + 0.4 Å.
1.5	Atoms are located to about + 0.1 Å.
0.77	Bond lengths in small crystals are measurable to 0.005 Å.

The significance of the X-ray crystallography in enzymology can be summarized, as follows:

(a) It provides detailed information about the arrangement of the atoms in the enzyme molecules.
(b) It aids in the structural elucidation of the active site of enzymes. It has been possible to detect the interactions that arise between

the enzyme and the substrate and to suggest therefrom what are the chemical origins of the catalytic effect.
(c) It aids in the investigation of enzyme mechanisms.

3.3.2 Groups of Enzyme Proteins

Over a thousand enzymes have now been described and over a hundred have been studied in great detail. Of these, about twenty have been analysed for three-dimensional structures by x-ray diffraction techniques. Three broad groups emerge.

(i) Monomeric Enzymes

These are enzymes with only one polypeptide chain in which the active site resides. Examples are lysozyme, (hen egg white), ribonuclease, papain, trypsin, carboxypeptidase.

(ii) Oligomeric Enzymes

This group contains at least two and as many as sixty or more subunits of firmly associated polypeptide chains to form the catalytically active enzyme protein. Examples are enolase (2 subunits); hexokinase (4 subunits); phosphorylase (4 subunits).

(iii) Multienzyme Complexes

This group consists of a number of enzymes engaged in a sequential series of reaction in the transformation of substrates to a product. They are usually tightly associated and each component catalyzes a distinct reaction. Examples include fatty acid synthetase, pyruvic acid dehydrogenase.

3.3.3 Enzyme Assemblages

The enzyme assemblages contain multiple enzyme activities and may be classified into two major types: (a) multienzyme complexes and (b) multifunctional enzymes.

(a) Multienzyme Complexes

These consist of non-covalently associated sub-units which catalyze one distinct and different reactions in a sequence. Examples include: pyruvate dehydrogenase complex which consist of 3 distinct enzymes, pyruvate decarboxylase (E_1), lipoate acetyltransferase (E_2) **and lipoamide dehydrogenase (E_3). The electron microscopy (EM) of the complex isolated from** *E. Coli* **revealed that there are 12 to 24 molecules of** E_1**; 12-24 molecules of E_2 and 8 trimers of E_3 constituting the core of the complex. These molecules had molecular weights as follows:** E_1; 1×10^5 daltons, E_2; 8×10^4 daltons and E_3; $5\text{-}6 \times 10^4$ daltons.

(b) Multifunctional Enzymes

These enzymes may or may not possess sub-units but each polypeptide chain has multiple catalytic functions. They are described as multiheaded, chimeric or polycephalic proteins whose binding sites are generated by folding of contiguous stretches of chains to yield autonomous domains.

Examples of these multifunctional enzymes include fatty acid synthetase complex, aspartokinase, homoserine dehydrogenase enzyme, tryptophan synthase enzyme.

3.3.4 Physiological Roles of Enzyme Assemblages

(i) They are highly efficient as compared to separable entities. They provide the greatest and closer interactions with substrates, due to increased local concentration within the catalytic sites.
(ii) The catalytic activities are restricted to a smaller region thus reducing the opportunities for intermediates to undergo competing reactions.
(iii) They provide an effective metabolic control.
(iv) The mutational effects are less minimised in multienzyme complexes due to existence of dynamic equilibrium between oligomeric and monomeric units of the system.
(v) They provide good targets for molecular evolution since any mutation causing a slight change in tertiary structure may be amplified through sub-unit interactions.

3.4 COENZYMES

Many enzymes which do catalyse a broad spectrum of reactions require the presence of a small non-protein 'prosthetic group' for efficient performance of catalytic function. They are more or less tightly linked to the protein and intimately concerned with the overall reaction. They are termed cofactors or coenzymes (Table 3.4) However, the term, "prosthetic group" is reserved for those molecules which are tightly bound to the enzyme. Coenzymes frequently contain structures not found in ordinary metabolites and behave as catalysts in the sense that they are eventually recovered in their original form. Therefore, they need not be present in high concentrations in the tissue any more than the apoenzyme need be.

So, the enzyme consists of the coenzyme and the associated polypeptide chains which are called the apoenzyme.

$$\text{Apoenzyme} + \text{Coenzyme} = \text{Enzyme}$$

It is important to note that many enzymes for which the biological function has been exactly established are known to be required because they are used to form vitamins. Examples include Vitamin B_6 - (pyridoxal, pyridoxamin; pyridoxine), Vitamin B_2 (thiamine pyrophosphate). (Figure 3.4 (c) and (d)).

Table 3.4: Examples of Important Co-Enzymes

Name of Coenzyme	Abbreviation	Function	Vitamin
1. Nicotinamide adenine dinucleotide	NAD, NADH (DPN, DPNH; CoI, CoIH$_2$)	Hydrogen transport	Niacinamide (B complex)
2. Nicotinamide adenine dinucleotide phosphate	NADP, NADPH (TPN, TPNH; CoII, CoIIH$_2$)	Hydrogen transport	Niacinamide (B complex)

3.	Flavin mononucleotide	(FMN)	Hydrogen transport	Riboflavin (Vitamin B_2)
4.	Flavin adenine dinucleotide	FAD	Hydrogen transport	Riboflavin (Vitamin B_2)
5.	Reduced glutathione	GSSG	Hydrogen transport	None
6.	Ascorbic Acid	-	Hydrogen transfer	Ascorbic acid (Vitamin C)
7.	Lipoic Acid (thioctic acid, reduced and oxidised)		Hydrogen transfer and acyl, succinyl group carrier. Acts in oxidative decarboxylation with TPP.	None
8.	Coenzyme A	CoA or CoA-SH	Acyl group carrier	Pantothenic acid
9.	Tetrahydrofolic acid CoF, THFA		Formyl group Folic acid transfer, hydroxy- methyl group transfer.	
10.	Pyrophosphothiamine TPP		Decarboxylation of Thiamine alpha keto acids. Forms (Vitamin B_1) an intermediate complex with the aldehyde.	

11.	Phosphopyridoxal PyP	Transamination and Pyridoxine decarboxylation. Schiff (Vitamin B_6) base formation as intermediate racemisation.
12.	Diphosphoglucose G-l, 6-dip (also glycerol 2,3diphosphate)*	Phosphate transfer None

The structural representations of some important coenzymes, cofactors, prosthetic groups and their derivatives are illustrated in Figure 3.4.

Nicotinamide Adenine Dinucleotide-reduced ($NADH_2$)

(a) NADP, $NADPH_2$ have ○ P at

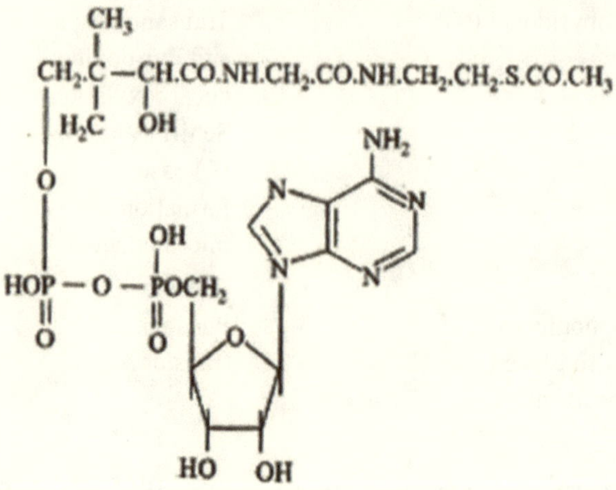

(b) Acetyl coenzyme A

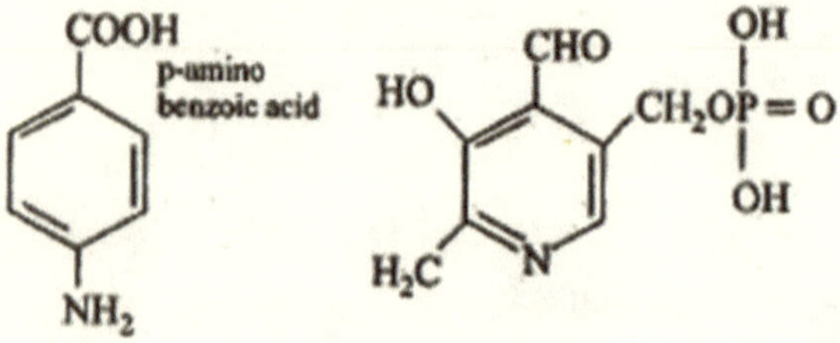

p-amino benzoic acid

(c) Pyridoxal phosphate

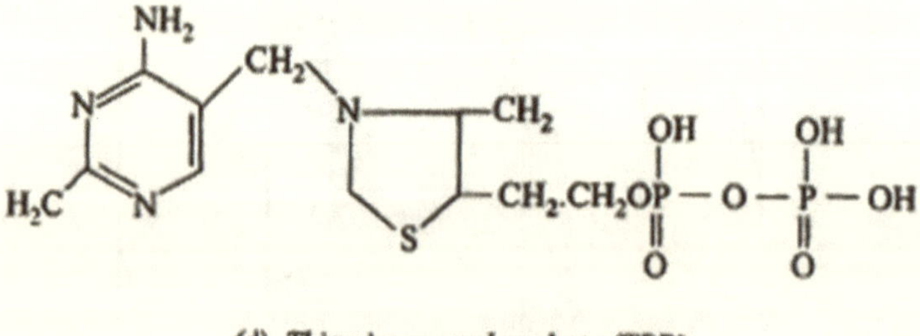

(d) Thiamine pyrophosphate (TPP)

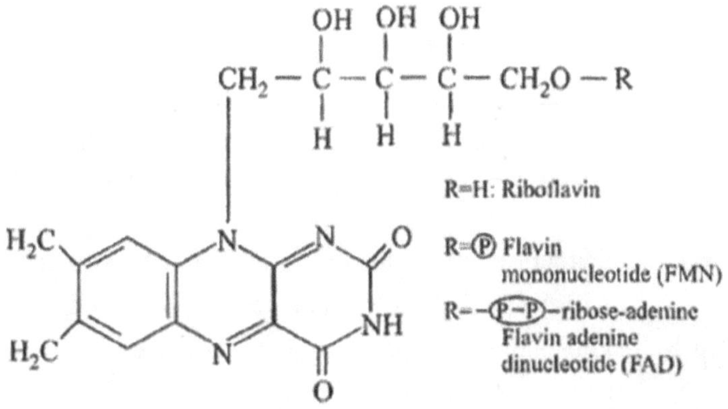

(e) *Riboflavin and derivatives*

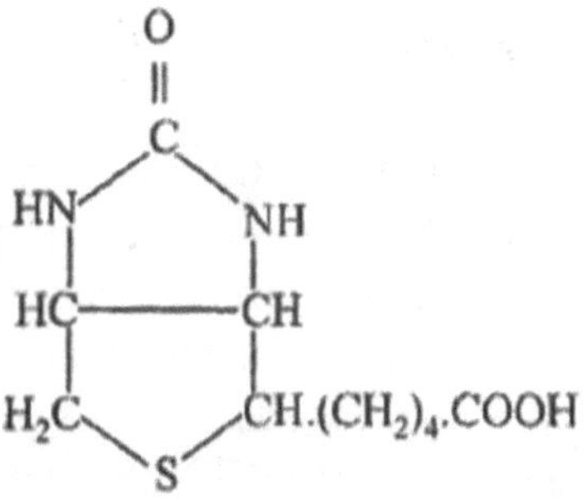

(f) *Biotin (vitamin H)*

Figure 3.4: Co-factors and prosthetic groups and their derivatives

Table 3.5: Some Enzymes Containing or
Requiring Metal Ions as Co-factors

Metal Ion	Enzymes
Zn^{2+}	Alcohol dehydrogenase, carboxypeptidase, Carbonic anhydrase.
Fe^{2+}/Fe^{+}	
Mn^{2+}	Cytochromes, Peroxidase, Catalase, Ferredoxin.
Mg^{2+}	Arginase; Phosphotransferases.
Cu^{2+} [Cu^{+}]	Phosphohydrolases; Phosphotransferases.
Na^{+}	Cytochrome oxidase, Tyrosinase.
K^{+}	Plasma membrane ATPase (also requires K^{+} and Mg^{2+}). Pyruvate phosphokinase (also requires Mg^{2+})

3.5 METALLOENZYMES

Many enzymes either contain tightly bound metal ions or require them for activity (Table 3.5). Those which contain a definite quantity of functional metal ions that is retained throughout purification are called *metalloenzymes;* whilst those which bind metal less tightly but require added metals for activity are referred to as **metal-activated enzymes.** The functions of these metal ions in enzyme catalysis have been studied by **X**-ray crystallography, magnetic resonance imaging (MRI) and electron spin resonance (ESR). The mechanism whereby metal ions perform their functions appear similar in metalloenzymes and metal activated enzymes.

3.5.1 Catalytic Function

The formation of ternary (3-component) complexes of the catalytic site, (Enz); a metal ion (M) and substrate (S) that exhibit 1:1:1 stoichiometry have been established. Four different kinds of complexes are possible therefrom; namely (I) substrate-bridge complex (Enz-S-M); (ii) Enzyme-bridge complex (M-Enz-S); (iii) Simple metal-bridge complex (Enz-M-S) and (iv) cyclic metal bridge complex.

All the four schemes are possible for the metal-activated enzymes. The metalloenzymes cannot form the [Enz-S-M], substrate-bridge complex because they retain the metal throughout purification, (i.e., are already as Enz-M).

The enzyme-bridge complexes, [M-Enz-S] are presumed to perform structural roles in maintaining an active conformation, (e.g, glutamine synthase) or to form a metal bridge to a substrate, (e.g. pyruvate kinase.)

The substrate-bridge complexes include the kinases (ATP-phosphotransferases). The reaction sequence exhibited by these enzymes which require nucleotide triphosphates is as follows:

$$ATP + M(H_2O)_6^2 \rightleftharpoons ATP - M(H_2O)_3^{2-} + 3H_2O \qquad (1)$$

$$ATP - M(H_2O)_3^{2-} + Enz \rightleftharpoons Enz - ATP - M(H_2O)_3^{2-} \qquad (2)$$

Invariably, the metal ions are thought to activate the phosphorus atoms and form a rigid polyphosphate-adenine complex of appropriate conformation in the active quartenary complex. In case of the metal-bridge complexes, the binary, Enz-M complex is the rate limiting step involving the departure of water from the co-ordination sphere of the metal ion.

$$Enz + M(H_2O)_6 \xrightarrow{Rapid} Enz+ - M(H_2O)_{6-n} + nH_2O$$

Rearrangement to active conformation (Enz$^+$); then follows:

$$Enz - M(H_2O)_{6-n} \xrightarrow{Slow} Enz^+ - M(H_2O)_{6-n}$$

Subsequently, the ternary metal-bridge complex is formed by the combination of the substrate (S) with the binary Enz-M complex, thus:

$$Enz - M + S \rightleftharpoons Enz - M - S \quad \text{or} \quad Enz{<}^{M}_{S}$$

Metal-bridge complexes

3.5.2 Physiological Roles

(a) The metal ions do participate in each of the four mechanisms by which enzymes are known to accelerate the rates of chemical reactions, namely

1. general acid-base catalysis,
2. covalent catalysis,
3. approximation of reactants, and
4. induction of strain in the enzyme or substrate.

(b) Metal ions are electrophiles (Lewis acids), and can share an electron pair forming a sigma bond. They may also be considered as "super acids" because they exist in neutral solutions frequently having a positive charge which is greater than unity.
(c) They can donate electrons that activate nucleophiles or act as nucleophiles themselves.
(d) Metals can serve as 3-dimensional templates for orientation of basic groups on the enzyme or substrate.

CHAPTER FOUR

Analytical Enzymology

4.0 INTRODUCTION

Enzymes are potentially valuable analytical reagents due to the following properties:

(a) high rates of catalysis which permit the rapid determination of activities in biological samples; leading to high rates of sample turnover. Hence, they have wide applications in the food industry and hospitals
(b) high specificity that permits the relatively easy detection and quantitation of small concentration of a metabolite or inhibitor in a crude mixture under mild conditions.

The main applications of analytical enzymology are as follows:

(i) Determination of enzyme mechanisms.
(ii) Quantitation of enzyme amounts.
(iii) Quantitation of metabolite, inhibitors and activators.
(iv) Structural investigation of cells, organelle and complex molecules.

4.1 MEASUREMENT OF ENZYME LEVELS

The level of an enzyme in a biological sample may be determined by measurement of either its catalytic activity or its molecular concentration. At saturating substrate concentration, an enzyme which obeys Michelis-Menten kinetics, the maximum rate, V, is $V = K_2 E$.

where K_2 = rate constant and E = total enzyme. Thus, it is possible to determine concentration, E, if either K_2 or V is known.

4.1.1 Units of Measurement

A frequent source of confusion is the use of variable arbitrary units to express enzymic activity. For example, there are seven different systems for expressing enzyme activity for the aspartate (AST) and alanine (ALT) amino-transferases (Table 4.1).

In practice, routine quantitative determination of enzymes are not feasible owing to the extreme difficulty of their isolation. Instead, enzyme activity is measured and this is suitable for clinical purposes. This requires optimal conditions in which the enzymes may function and thus attention is paid especially to temperature, pH of the medium, amount of enzyme concentrations or substrates and presence of activators or inhibitors.

When the appropriate conditions are assembled, the rate of reaction catalysed by the enzyme is measured. The most convenient are the so-called reactions of *zero order* in which the measured rate is proportionate to the quantity of enzyme present (when the reaction time is doubled, the amount of product is also doubled).

The situations when these conditions are fulfilled are infrequent, and catalytic activities are usually compared not by reference to a primary standard measurement equivalent to molarity, but by the use of the empirical and relative quantities called **International Units** or *Katals*.

Table 4.1: Comparison of activities of "AST" and "ALT" expressed in arbitrary units

Unit	AST' (Aspartate Transaminase)		ALT' (Alanine Transaminase)	
	Range	Mean	Range	Mean
Karmen	9-32	19.6	-	-
Wroblewski,	-	-	1-56	16
Steinberg	10-33	16	-	-
Baron	8-25	16	-	-
Bowers	16-44	25	6-75	22
Caband	4-40	16.4	-	-
King	23-107	16.5	22-110	54.7

The Enzyme Commission of the International Union of Biochemistry appreciating the situation, recommended the use of a Standard Unit (U) known as the International Unit (I.U.).

Data which are expressed in international units are comparable solely when identical substrates, amount of buffer solutions, pH values, temperature, activators, times and serum fractions have been used. This means that only under identical fractions have been used. That is, identical values can only be obtained with identical condition. Modifications, no matter how small, of defined methods will lead to different results, even when expressed in International Units.

4.2 DEFINITIONS OF ENZYME ACTIVITY PARAMETERS

(i) *International Unit* (I.U.) is defined as the amount of enzyme that will catalyse the transformation of one micromole of substrate per minute under standard conditions.
(ii) *Katal* (Kat) is the amount of activity that converts one mole of substrate to product per second, thus 1 katal = $10^6/60$ I.U.
(iii) *Specific Activity* refers to activity/mass; or Katals/ kilogram of protein. It is also expressed as I.U./protein.
(iv) *Concentration of Enzyme Activity* is expressed as activity/ volume or Katals/litre or I.U. /litre

(v) *Catalytic Constant* = $\dfrac{\text{moles of product per minute}}{\text{mole of pure enzyme}}$

(vi) *Turnover Number* = $\dfrac{\text{Catalytic constant}}{\text{Number of active sites}}$

4.3 MEASUREMENT OF CATALYTIC ACTIVITY

Catalytic activity of an enzyme is measured in terms of the rate of the reaction catalysed. The reaction rate has now been expressed in *Units* of μmol/min - (International Units). According to the SI system, the unit **of** *mol/s.* This kind of quantity is called *katal* (k, cat). Hence

$$IU \equiv 16.67 \times 10^{-9} \text{ kat} = 16.67 \text{ ηkcat}.$$

This unit does not agree with the definition of the reaction rate in classical reaction kinetics, where the measured magnitude is the change in **concentration per unit time:** here it is change in **amount per unit time.**

4.3.1 Experimental Consideration

In practice, for example, in photometric determination, one always measures time-dependent changes in concentrations {mol/l.s. from $\Delta A/\Delta t$}; the change in amount per unit time (mol/s) can be via the volume, in order to obtain IU or *kat*.

(i) Thus, for measurement of the catalytic activity, Z, of enzymes, the rate of the catalysed reaction is used, the substrate conversion per time unit or mol/s.

From Lambert-Beer Law,

$$c = \dfrac{\log I_0/I}{\varepsilon \times d} = \dfrac{A}{\varepsilon \times d} \text{ mmol/L}$$

For chemical reactions, this gives

$$c_1 - c_2 = \frac{A_1 - A_2}{\varepsilon \times d}; \quad \Delta c = \frac{\Delta A}{\varepsilon \times d} \text{ (mmol/L)}.$$

With complete conversion ($c_2 = 0$) it is

$$c = \frac{\Delta A}{\varepsilon \times d} \text{ mmol/L} \qquad \text{(in the cuvette)}.$$

(ii) For the determination of the concentration of the sample the ratio of total volume to the sample volume (V:v) is to be considered. Hence

$$c = \frac{\Delta A \times V}{\varepsilon \times d \times v} \text{ (mmol/L)} \qquad \text{(in the sample)}$$

and

$$c = \frac{\Delta A \times V \times MW}{\varepsilon \times d \times v} \qquad \text{(in the sample)}$$

Therefore in the case of enzyme-catalyzed reaction;

(i) **Catalytic activity, Z,**

$$Z = \frac{c \times V}{\Delta t} = \frac{\Delta A \times V}{1000 \times \varepsilon \times d \, \Delta t}$$

[Units: $l \times mmol^{-1} \times mm^{-1}$; V, (assay volume) in litre, d (in minutes) and t (in seconds)]

or

$$Z = \frac{\Delta c \times V}{\Delta t} = \frac{\Delta A \times V \times 1000 \, \mu mol/min}{\varepsilon \times d \times \Delta t} \quad \ldots(U)$$

Symbols

ε = absorption coefficient; litre × mmol $^{-1}$ × mm $^{-1}$
A = absorbance
ΔA = absorbance change
V = assay volume, (litre)
v = volume of sample used in assay, (litre)
t = time, (seconds)
Δt = interval between measurements, (seconds)
d = light path, (mm).
c = concentration of substance, (mols/litre; g/litre)
z = catalytic activity; (U, kat)
MW = wt of one millimole or mg/mmole.
b = catalytic activity concentration; IU/Litre, kat/litre.

(ii) **Catalytic activity concentration (kat/litre):**

$$b = \frac{\Delta A \times V}{1000 \times \varepsilon \times d \times \Delta t \times v} \text{ mols/} \times \text{litre}$$

or

Catalytic activity concentration

$$= \frac{\Delta A \times V \times 1000}{\varepsilon \times d \times \Delta t \times v} \;\mu mol/min \times litre \quad \ldots u/L$$

(iii) Catalytic activity related to the mass of protein; (*Specific Activity*), that is,

$$\frac{\text{Specific activity}}{(kat/g)} = \frac{\Delta A \times V}{1000 \times \varepsilon \times d \times \Delta t \times v \times c \text{ protein}}$$

or

$$\frac{\text{Specific activity}}{(U/g)} = \frac{\Delta A \times V \times 1000}{\varepsilon \times d \times \Delta t \times v \times c \text{ protein}} \ldots$$

4.4 ASSAY TECHNIQUES FOR ENZYME ACTIVITY

In any kinetic study, the essential element is the availability of convenient assays for measuring either the rate of formation of products or the rate of depletion of substrates. The classical procedures are manometry, viscometry and polarimetry. The modern techniques, namely Nuclear Magnetic Resonance, (NMR), Electron Spin Resonance (ESR) are now gaining popularity. However, the common procedures, namely spectrophotometry, spectrofluorometry, automatic titrations and radiometry are still in routine use. The parameters to which each technique has been associated are listed as shown in Table 4.2.

Table 4.2: Techniques for the determination of enzyme activity or concentration of metabolites (products)

Parameter	Measuring Technique	Example
Extinction	Photometry	Dehydrogenases, (NADH),
Fluorescence	Fluorimetry	(NADH)"
Isotope content	Radiometry	Nucleases
PH	Titration	Trypsin
Heat	Calorimetry	Glucose
O_2 content	Polarimetry	Glucose

We shall discuss some of these techniques briefly.

4.4.1 Spectrophotometry

Many substances absorb light in the ultraviolet or visible regions of the spectrum. Accordingly, the Lambert-Beer's Law:

$$A = \log\frac{I_0}{I} = \varepsilon CL$$

where I_0 is the intensity of incident light, I is the intensity of transmitted light, ε is the absorption or extinction coefficient, C is the concentration of the absorbing substances in moles/litres and L is the light path length.

This equation enables us to calculate the concentration or the extinction coefficient (ε).

Spectrophotometry is particularly useful with naturally occurring chromophores. For example the activities of many dehydrogenases may be measured from the rates of disappearance of NADH (reduced nicotinamide adenine dinucleotide) at 340 nm ($\varepsilon = 6.23 \times 10^3$ m^{-1} cm^{-1}); since NAD does not absorb at this wavelength. In some cases artificial substrates may be used, for example p-nitrophenylesters are good substrates for esterases. The p-nitrophenolate ion absorbs at 420 nm. ($\varepsilon = 1.1 \times 10^4$ m^{-1} cm^{-1}). The sensitivity of the method depends on the magnitude of the extinction coefficient.

4.4.2 Spectrofluorometry

Some compounds absorb light and then re-emit it as a longer wavelength. This is known as fluorescence. The process occurs by a photon being absorbed by a compound to give an excited state, whose half-life approximately, (10 ns) then decays by re-emission of a photon. The decay may take place by a collision with another ion or transfer of energy to another group; hence the fluorescence is then said to be quenched. The intensity of the fluorescent light is proportional to the intensity of the exciting beam. The efficiency of the process is termed quantum yield, q, which is given by the ratio:

$$q = \frac{\text{number of quanta emitted}}{\text{number of quanta absorbed}}$$

Generally, q is always less than 1.

The natural fluorophores include NADH, tryptophan, tyrosine. Fluorescent synthetic substrates for esterases, phosphatases, sulphatases and glycosidases contain 4 methylumbelliferron, a highly fluorescent derivative of phenol.

4.4.3 Automatic Titration Methods

This technique is applicable for hydrolytic reactions where proton release may be followed by titration with a base.

This is best done by use of the pH-stat equipment. In this equipment, a glass electrode registers the pH of the solution which is kept constant by the automatic addition of base from a syringe controlled by an electronic circuit. The limit of detection is approximately 50 nonamoles. The reaction volumes of roughly one millimeter can be employed in such assays.

4.4.4 Radiometry

It is the most sensitive assay method which involves the use of radioactively-labelled substrates. Radioactivity is measured in curies (Ci) which is equivalent to 2.2×10^{12} dpm (disintegration per minute). The common isotopes are 3_H, 32_P, 35_S and 14_C. These emit β-electrons. The principle of this technique is that one of the substrates participating in the reaction is used in a radioactively-labelled form. The reaction leads to a specifically-labelled product.

4.5 FACTORS AFFECTING ENZYME ACTIVITY

The standard methods for the determination of enzyme activity require optimum experimental conditions. These conditions relate to the nature and concentration of all reactants, the pH and the ionic strength of the buffer and other parameters. We shall now discuss the most important briefly.

4.5.1 Temperature

Like all chemical reactions, enzyme catalysed reactions are sensitive to temperature changes. The temperature coefficient of the reaction rate can be as large as 10% per degree or more. This means that for a temperature rise of 1 °C, the value found for the catalytic activity of an enzyme is about 10% too high. The temperature dependence on chemical reaction can be formulated mathematically. Arrhenius found empirically that a linear relation generally exists between the logarithm of the rate constant k, and the reciprocal of the absolute temperature, T. Thus,

$$\ln k = \ln A - \frac{B}{T},$$

where T = absolute temperature, A and B are constants. But

$$B = \frac{E_A}{R}$$

$$A = PZ$$

where E_A is the Arrhenius Activation Energy, R is the Gas constant, P the Steric Factor and Z is the Collision Efficiency,

$$\log_{10} k = \log Z - \frac{E_A}{2.303} \times \frac{1}{RT}$$

By means of Arrhenius plot, that is, plot of log k against $\frac{1}{T}$ one can determine, for a given enzyme reaction, the activation energy of the reaction. The effects of temperature on rate constant was described by empirical Arrhenius equation,

$$E_A = RT^2 \frac{d \ln k}{dT}$$

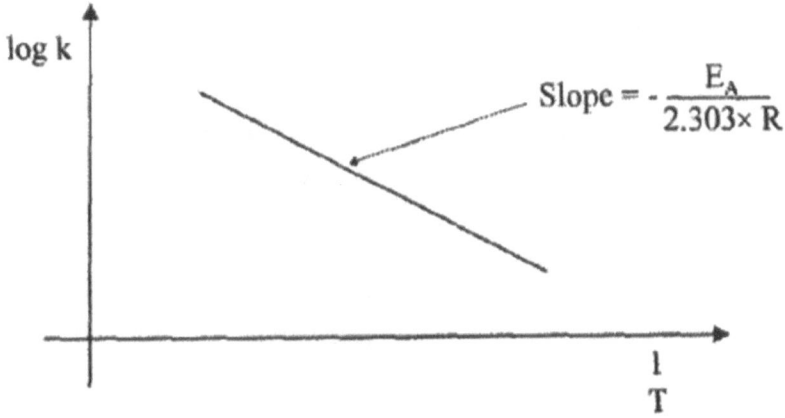

Figure 4.1: Temperature dependence of rate constants. (The Arrhenius plot)

4.5.2 Effect of pH on Enzyme Activity

The hydrogen ion concentration affects the affinity of an enzyme for its substrate, the maximum rate of reaction, and the protein stability. The resultant of these effects gives generally a narrow pH range with activity profile with an optimum. The effects of pH on macromolecular stability of the enzyme can be quantitated by exposing it to different hydrogen ion concentration for varying times and followed by assay at a fixed value.

Interpreting the observed pH-rate profiles in terms of side chain ionisation at the active site; gives a bell-shaped curve. This can be treated as the composite of two sigmoidal titration curves, Figure 4.2.

When allowance is made for any protonic dissociation constants pertinent to the substrate alone. These two types of pH activity profiles are commonly referred to as bell-shaped and sigmoid shaped curves.

The binding of substrate to enzyme site is itself pH dependent due to changes in the detailed conformation of the site or to the pH-dependent charges of the enzyme protein.

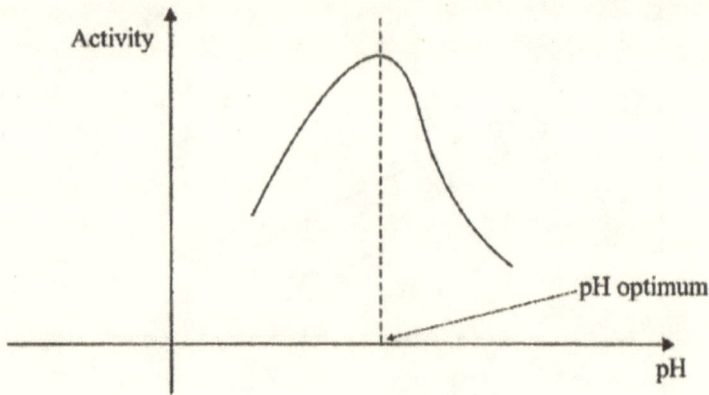

Figure 4.2: Typical pH rate profile of enzyme catalysed reaction

The latter is more profound with substrate which are themselves charged.

The effect of pH on enzyme activity can often be accounted for on the basis of the two catalytic models. Hence

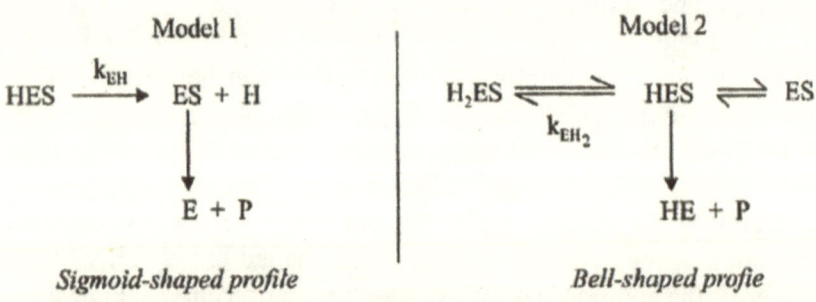

In the process of fitting experimental profile of pH versus maximal activity to the appropriate models, the dissociation constant k_{EH_1} and k_{EH_2} are determined.

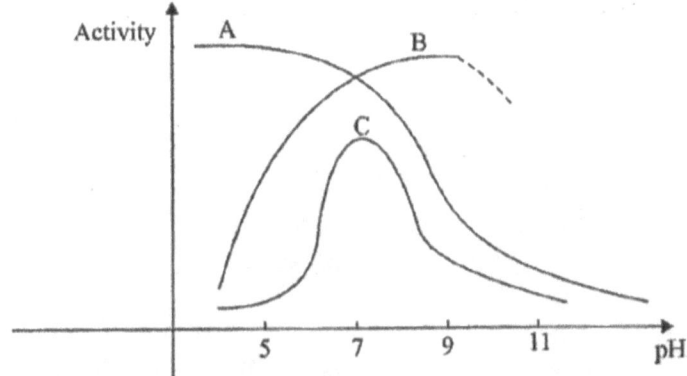

Figure 4.3: Typical variations in enzyme activity as a function of pH of the medium

Quantitative Treatment on Effect of pH on Enzyme Activity

From the schematic representation of effects of pH on the reaction parameters, the following assumptions can be made:

(i) Michael-Menten Henri mechanism is followed in which the breakdown of E-S complex (k_2) is rate-limiting.
(ii) Catalysis depends only on two ionisations at the active site with their rates of ionisation rapid compared to the rate of the catalytic process.
(iii) Rates of formation and breakdown of EHS are faster than that of ES or EH2S, i.e

$$V = k_2 EH_2 S$$

Based on these assumption, the scheme is subjected to steady state analysis.

REVIEW QUESTIONS

1. Describe fully the experimental procedure for the isolation and purification of a **named** enzyme. State FOUR parameters by which one can characterize this enzyme.
2. State the various types of conformations that can be found associated with an enzyme molecule.
3. Describe briefly how the tertiary structure of an enzyme relates to its biological function.
4. Discuss concisely the contribution of X-ray crystallographic studies in the field of Enzymology. Illustrate your answer with specific named enzymes.
5. Write notes on
   - Isomorphous Replacement
   - Secondary Structures of Enzymes
   - Enzyme Assemblages
   - Metalloenzymes
   - Multi-enzyme complexes
   - Effect of pH on enzyme activity

REFERENCES

A. HISTORY OF ENZYMOLOGY.

1. Payen, A & Persoz J.F. (1833). **Ann. Chim. Phys.** 53 73-92
2. Berzelivs, J.J. (1837) **Lehrbuch der chemie, 3, Auflage.** Vol 6 19-25 Arnold, Dresden.
3. Pasteur, L. (1860). "De l' origine des ferments. Nouvelle experience relatives aux generations dikes spontanees". **C.R. Acad. Sci**
4. Liebig, J. (1839). **Liebigs. Ann. Chem. Pharm.** 30. 250-288
5. Kuhne, W. (1877). **Verh. Naturh. Med. Verein** Heidelberg N.F.I. 194-198.
6. Summer, J.B. (1926). **J. Biol. Chem.** 69. 435.
7. Schwann, T. (1837). **Liebigs. Ann. Chem. Pharm.** 41, 184-193
8. Liebig, J. & Wahler, F. (1837). **Ann. Chem. Pharm.** 22, 1.
9. Fourcroy, A.F. & Vaugelin. N.T. (1799). *Ann. Chem.* 31, 48-71.
10. Kuhne. W. (1866/8) **Lehrbuch der physiologischen Chemie,** W. Engelmann, Leipzig.

11. **Eberle. J.N. (1834).** *Physiologie der Vergaung nach Versuchen auf naturlichen und Kunstlichem* **Wege Wurzburg**
12. Kirchhoff, C.G.S. (1814). *J. fur Chem* U *Physik.* 14, 389-398.
13. Nothrop. J.H. (1930). *J. Gen. Physiol.* 13, 739-766.
14. Northrop. J.H. (1932). "Story of isolation of crystalline pepsin and trypsin". *Scientific Monthly* 35, 333-340
15. Robiquet, P.J. & Boutron-Chalard, A.F. (1830). *Ann. Chim. Phys.* 44, 352.
16. Dubrunfaut, A.P. (1846). *Ann. Chim.* 3me ser. 18, 99-108.
17. Berthelot M. (1860). *C.R. Acad. Sci.* (Paris) 50, 980-984.
18. Musculus, F.A. (1876). *C.R. Acad. Sci.* (Paris) 82, 334.
19. **Corvisart, L. (1857).** *Collection de memoires sur une fonction peu connue du pancrease, la digestion des ailments azotes.* **Par.**
20. Northrop, J.H. & Kunitz, M. (1931). *Science* 73, 262, cf i.c. (84)
21. **Hughes, G. (1750)** *Natural History of Barbados.*
22. Wurtz A. & Bouchut, E. (1879). *C.R. Acad. Sci.* (Paris) 89, 425.
23. Balls, A.K. & Lineweaver, H. (1939) *J. Biol. Chem.* 130, 669-686.
24. Sumner: (1926). *J. Biol. Chem.* 69: 435,
25. Sumner: (1928). *J. Biol. Chem.* 76: 149.
26. Sumner, J.B. & Dounce, A.L. (1937). *J. Biol. Chem.* 121, 417-424.
27. Sumner, J.B. & Dounce, A.L. (1939). *J. Biol. Chem.* 127, 439-447.
28. Dounce, A.L. *et al.* (1978). *Arch. Biochem. Biophys.* 181, 251-265.
29. Dounce, A.L. & Allen, P.Z. (1987). *Arch. Biochem. Biophys.* 275, 13-16.
30. Theorell, A.H.T. (1976). *Trends. Biochem. Sci.* 1. 45
31. Fruton, J.S. (1977). *Trends Bioch. Sci.* 2, 210-211.
32. Dounce, A.L. Leggo, C.T. Voltmer, A & Chanda, S.K. (1974). *Biochim. Biophys.* 342, 81-88.
33. Commission on Biochemical Nomenclature (1973); "1972
34. **Boyer, P.D., Lardy, H and Myrback. K. (1959).** *The Enzymes - Academic Press. Recommendations Biochemical Nomenclature.* **Elsevier Amsterdam.**
35. **Laidler (1954).** *Introduction to the Chemistry of Enzymes.*
36. Alberty; R.A. (1953). *J. Amer. Chem. Sci.* 75, 1928-1932

37. Lineweaver, H and Burk D. (1934). *J. Amer. Chem. Soc.* 56. 658-666. B. quoted by Haldane J.B.S. & Stern. K.G. (1932) Allegemeine Chemic der Enzymes.

B. STRUCTURE OF ENZYMES

Lewitt, M. & Chotia, C. (1976). "Structure Patterns in globular proteins". *Nature* (Lond), 261: 552-556.

Richards, F.M. (1974). "The interpretation of protein structure. Total volume, group volume, distribution and pacing". *J. Mol. Biol.*, 82; 1-14

Crothia, C. (1975) Structure invariants in protein foldings. Nature (Lond), 254: 307-308

Moult, J., Tomath, A. *et al.* (1976). "The structure of triclinic lysozyme at 2-5 A resolution". *J. Mol Biol.* 100, 179-195.

Blake, C.C.F. & Johnson, L.N. (1984). "Trends in Biochem". *Sci.* 9, 4. 147-151 Protein Structure (1976)

C. SUGGESTIONS FOR FURTHER READING

(i) **X-ray analysis and Protein Structure:** P.H. Crick, and Kendrew F.C. (1957). *Adv. in protein chemistry* 12 pp 133-214

(ii) **Structure of Hen-Egg White Lysozyme: Three-dimensional fourier synthesis at 2 Å resolution.** Blake, C. C. F, Koenig, A. ET AL., (1965). NATURE 206, 4986, 757-763

(iii) **Structure of Hemoglobin: A three-dimensional fourier synthesis of reduced human Hb. At 5.5 Å resolution.** Muirhead & Perutz, M. (1963). NATURE, Vol. 199. 633-639.

(iv) **Relation between structure & sequence of Hemoglobin:** Perutz, M.L. (1962). NATURE, Vol. 194, 914-911

(v) **The three-dimensional sturcture of a protein molecule:** Kendrew, J.C (1961). SCIENTIFIC AMERICAN, DEC.

(vi) **The three-dimensional structure of an enzyme molecule:** Phillips, D.C. (1966). SCIENTIFIC AMERICAN, Vol. 215, 78-90

(vii) **The Haemoglobin molecule:** Perutz, M.F. (1964). *Scientific American,* Nov.

PART II

Enzyme Kinetics

CHAPTER FIVE

Enzyme Kinetics I

5.0 INTRODUCTION TO ENZYME KINETICS

General Consideration

Kinetics is the study of reaction rates and the factors influencing them. All kinetics work is based on the *law of mass action* which states that the rate of reaction is proportional to the product of the activities of each reactant; each activity being raised to the power of the number of molecules of that reactant taking part. Thus, this can be illustrated by the reaction equation below.

$$aA + bB \rightarrow \text{Products}$$

Rate of reaction = (activity of A)^a × (activity of B)^b

For practical purposes, the term "activity" is usually replaced by concentration.

5.1 ORDER OF REACTIONS

There are three major types of order of reactions often encountered generally in enzyme kinetics.

(i) Zero-Order Reaction

The rate of reaction is independent of the concentration of any reactant.

(ii) First Order Reaction

The rate is proportional to the concentration of one reactant. For example, consider the reaction: A → P

$$\text{Rate, } V = -\frac{d[A]}{dt} = \frac{d[P]}{dt}$$

$$V = k[A]$$

$$-\frac{dA}{dt} = \text{rate of decrease of reactant A,}$$

$$\frac{dP}{dt} = \text{rate of formation of product P.}$$

The rate side has a function containing (A) to the first power and the reaction is therefore said to be first order in (A). The proportionally constant, k is called the rate constant (or coefficient or specific reaction rate). It has the dimension of time $^{-1}$.

(iii) Second Order Reaction

The rate is proportional to the concentration of the two reactants or to the second power of a single reactant.

Consider the reaction:

(i) A + B → P + (Q) + ...
The rate equation is given by

$$\text{Rate, } V = -\frac{d[A]}{dt} = -\frac{d[B]}{dt} = +\frac{d[P]}{dt} = k[A][B]$$
$$= k[A][B].$$

ESSENTIALS OF ENZYMOLOGY

This reaction is second-order overall for its rate is proportional to the product of two concentration terms (those of A and B respectively).

The rate constant k, in this instance, has the dimension of concentration^{-1} time $^{-1}$.

(ii) For a special case: 2A $\rightarrow$ P
Rate equation:

$$V = -\frac{d[A]}{dt} = +\frac{d[P]}{dt} = k[A]^2$$

This form of the equation is also obeyed if we start with identical concentrations of A and B.

5.2 GENERAL RATE EQUATIONS FOR FIRST ORDER REACTIONS

The rate of a first order reaction is directly proportional to the concentration of one of the reacting species only. For example, consider the reaction:

$$A \rightarrow P \text{ (products)}$$

The rate equation is given by:

$$\frac{dx}{dt} = k(a - x). \qquad (1)$$

The constant, k used in (1) is known as the *first order rate constant*. 'a' denotes the initial concentration of A and x is the concentration of the product, P, formed at time 't'. Equation (1) may be written as

$$\frac{dx}{(a-x)} = kdt$$

and on integrating we find an equation from which a value for the first order rate constant can be obtained. Thus,

$$-\ln(a-x) = kt + c \qquad (2)$$

where c is a constant. To find the value of c, we require related values of t and x. Thus, when t = 0, x must also be zero,

$$\therefore c = \ln a.$$

Consequently, we can write

$$kt = \ln a - \ln(a-x).$$

On re-arranging, this equation yields k in terms of a, x and t:

$$kt = \ln \frac{a}{(a-x)}$$

$$k = \frac{\ln \frac{a}{(a-x)}}{t} = 2.303 \frac{\ln \frac{a}{(a-x)}}{t} \qquad (3)$$

This last equation may be written in the form of the general equation for a straight line, y = mx + c:

$$\log(a-x) = -(k/2.303)t + \log a, \qquad (4)$$

which allows some appreciation of graphical methods of data presentation for first order reactions.

5.3 GENERAL RATE EQUATION FOR SECOND ORDER REACTIONS

The rate of second order reaction is proportional to the product of two concentration terms. For the general case of a reaction between two species, A and B, such that:

$$A + B \rightarrow \text{Products}$$

The rate of reaction will be given by

$$\frac{dx}{dt} = k(a-x)(b-x), \qquad (5)$$

since the coefficients and exponents are equal to unity. In equation (5), the rate constant k will be a second order rate constant. In certain cases, equation (5) can be simplified.

Thus, when a = b or when the species A and B are identical, equation (5) becomes:

$$\frac{dx}{dt} = k(a-x)^2, \qquad (6)$$

Thus,

$$\frac{dx}{(a-x)^2} = k\,dt.$$

On integrating, this becomes

$$\frac{1}{(a-x)} = kt + c \qquad (7)$$

where c is a constant. The value of c can be found by using related values of t and x. Thus, when t = 0 and x = 0 then c becomes 1/a, hence, we can write:

$$\frac{1}{(a-x)} = kt + \frac{1}{a} \qquad (8)$$

from which, it can be seen that the second order rate constant, *k, will possess* units *of* reciprocal *time and* reciprocal concentration.

5.4 DERIVATION OF MICHAELIS-MENTEN EQUATION

The theory of enzyme catalysis assumes that the enzyme first forms a complex with its substrate; this complex subsequently breaks down, giving the free enzyme and the products of the reaction.

$$E + S \underset{k_{-1}}{\overset{k_1 \quad K_S}{\rightleftharpoons}} ES \xrightarrow{k_2} E + P$$

enzyme + substrate   (enzyme – substrate)   product
                                   complex

(9)

k_1, k_{-1}, k_2 denote rate constants.

The formation of enzyme-substrate complex as an intermediate in the reaction (equation (9)) above, provides an explanation for the saturating effect of increasing substrate concentration in enzyme catalysis. Michaelis and Menten derived a general equation for the relationship between reaction velocity and substrate concentration. The mathematical expression which also described the observed hyperbolic dependence of initial velocity on substrate concentration (Figure 6.0) was developed from the following assumptions:

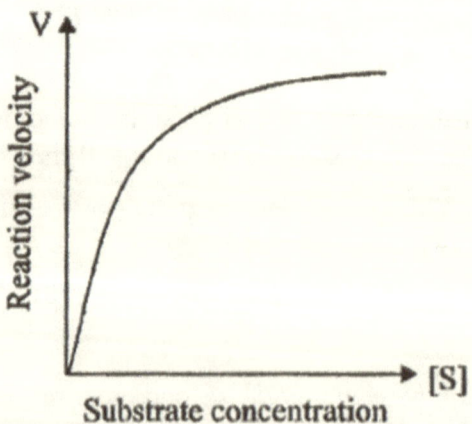

Figure 5.1: Dependence of reaction velocity, V, over substrate concentration [S] in an enzyme-catalysed reaction

(a) The enzyme-substrate complex is in equilibrium with the free enzyme species in solution and
(b) Only by means of this complex could products be formed at an observable rate.

Hence, the mechanism can be represented as follows:

$E + S \rightleftharpoons ES$ (Equilibrium formation of the enzyme- substrate complex) (10)

$ES \rightleftharpoons E + P$. (breakdown of complex to products with regeneration of enzyme) (11)

The equilibrium reaction (6.2) can be described by an apparent equilibrium constant, K_s defined as:

$$K_s = \frac{[E][S]}{[ES]} \quad (12)$$

where [E] and [S] are the free concentrations of enzyme and substrate respectively and [ES] in the concentration of enzyme-substrate complex.

The rate of product formation, V, is given by

$$V = K_{cat}[S] \quad (13)$$

Where, K_{cat} is the first order rate constant for the breakdown of the enzyme-substrate complex and V, initial velocity. When the substrate concentrations are high compared to the catalytic concentrations of enzyme, the free concentration of enzyme will be substantially decreased but that of the substrate not significantly. The free enzyme, [E], is given as:

$$[E] = [E_0] - [ES]$$

Substituting for K_s in (6.4)

$$K_s = \frac{\{E_0 - ES\}S_0}{ES}$$

$$\therefore [ES] = \frac{[E_0]S}{K_s + S_0} \qquad (14)$$

where E_0 and S_0 are total initial concentrations. On substituting for [ES] in equation (13) we find,

$$V = \frac{K_{cat} E_0 \cdot S_0}{K_s + S_0} \qquad (15)$$

The maximum velocity is attained when all enzyme molecules are saturated with substrate. Hence,

$$V_{max} = K_{cat} \cdot E_0$$

$$\therefore V = \frac{V_{max} \cdot S_0}{K_s + S_0} \qquad (16)$$

Equation (16) is known as the ***"Michaelis-Menten Equation"***. At low substrate concentration, $K_s > S_0$, therefore,

$$V = \frac{V_{max} \cdot S_0}{K_s} \qquad (17)$$

that is, the initial velocity increases linearly with the substrate concentration. Conversely, at high substrate concentration, or saturating substrate concentration; $S_0 > K_s$, thus,

$$V = V_{max} \qquad (18)$$

that is, the initial rate will approach the maximum velocity, the limiting value termed, V_{max}. The concentration of substrate at which

$V = \dfrac{1}{2} V_{max}$ is termed Km, (*Michaelis Constant*)

The term, K_m is called the Michaelis constant, which is equivalent to the substrate concentration that yields half-maximal velocity. It is a constant for a given enzyme, and its numerical value provides a means of comparing enzymes from different organisms or from different tissues of the same organism; or from the same tissue at different stages of development.

The Michaelis constant indicates the relative 'suitability' of alternate substrates of a particular enzyme. That is, the substrate with the lowest K_m value has the highest apparent affinity for the enzyme. (hence, the 'best' substrate is that which has the highest $\dfrac{V_{max}}{K_m}$ ratio).

5.5 DETERMINATION OF THE KINETIC CONSTANTS, V_{max}, K_m

The direct plot of initial velocity 'V' versus substrate concentration is a hyperbola; thus, it is rather difficult to determine Vmax, and hence the substrate concentration that yields $\dfrac{1}{2}V_{max}$ (i.e. K_m). Therefore, the determination of the kinetic constants is best carried out by plotting the data in one of the linear forms as described below.

5.6.1 Lineweaver-Burke (Double-reciprocal plot) Plot

This is based on the rearrangement of the Henri-Michaelis-Menten equation into a linear form similar to simple equation y = mx + c which represents a straight line.

On rearranging equation (16) we find,

$$\frac{V}{V_{max}} = \frac{[S]}{K_m + S} \quad (19).$$

On inverting, we obtain

$$\frac{V_{max}}{V} = \frac{K_m + [S]}{[S]} \quad (20)$$

If equation (20) is rearranged,

$$\frac{1}{V} = \frac{K_m}{V_{max}[S]} + \frac{[S]}{V_{max}[S]} \quad (21)$$

or

$$\frac{1}{V} = \frac{K_m}{V_{max}} \cdot \frac{1}{[S]} + \frac{1}{V_{max}} \quad (22)$$

Therefore, a plot of $\frac{1}{V}$ against $\frac{1}{[S]}$ proposed by Lineweaver-Burke, gives a straight line rather than a *hyperbola.*

Slope = $\frac{K_m}{V_{max}}$ and the *Intercept* on the Y-axis = $\frac{1}{V_{max}}$

But when $\frac{1}{V} = 0$; then $\frac{1}{[S]} = -\frac{1}{K_m}$.

Thus, the intercept on the $\frac{1}{[S]}$ is $-\frac{1}{K_m}$ [Figure 5.2].

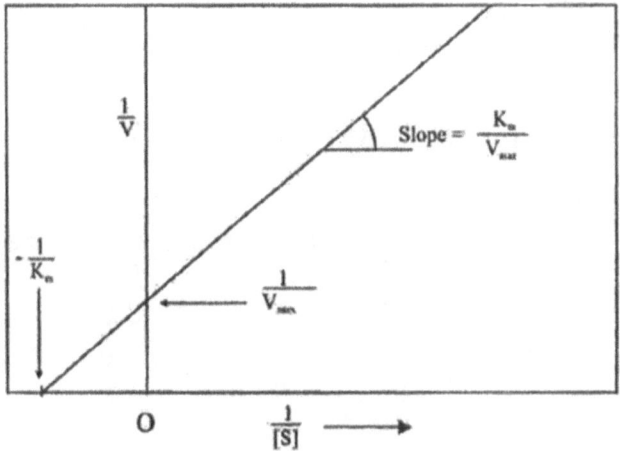

Figure 5.2: *The Lineweaver-Burk plot*

5.6.2 Hanes-Woolf Plot

This is a plot of [S]/V versus [S]. The Lineweaver – Burk equation may be rearranged to yield the linear equation, for the Hanes-Woolf plot.

L-B Equation:

$$\frac{1}{V} = \frac{K_m}{V_{max}} \frac{1}{[S]} + \frac{1}{V_{max}}$$

Multiplying each side of equation (22) by [S] yields

$$\frac{[S]}{V} = \frac{[S] K_m}{V_{max} [S]} + \frac{[S]}{V_{max}}$$

or

$$\frac{[S]}{V} = \frac{1}{V_{max}} [S] + \frac{K_m}{V_{max}} \quad (23)$$

Thus, a plot of $\frac{[S]}{V}$ versus [S] is linear with a slope of $\frac{1}{V_{max}}$.

The intercept on the $\frac{[S]}{V}$ -axis is $\frac{K_m}{V_{max}}$.

When $\frac{[S]}{V} = 0$, the intercept on the [S]-axis is K_m; (Figure 5.3).

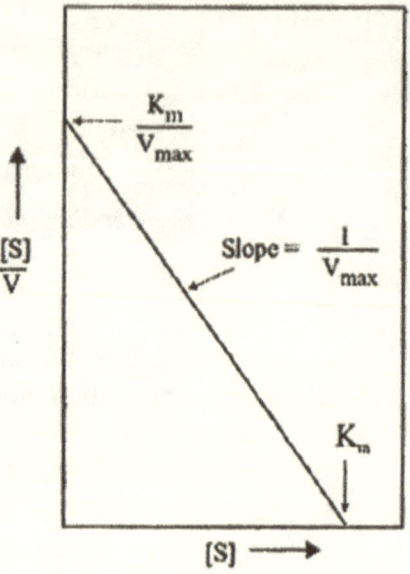

Figure 5.3: The Hanes-Woolf plot

5.6.3. The Eadie-Hofstee Plot: *(single-reciprocal plot)*

The Michaelis-Menten equation (equation 16) can be rearranged as described above for this single reciprocal plot $\frac{V}{[S]}$ versus V. On rearranging equation (19), we find

$$V_{max} = \frac{VK_m}{[S]} + V \qquad (24)$$

When both sides of equation (24) are divided by K_m it becomes

$$\frac{V_{max}}{K_m} = \frac{V}{[S]} + \frac{V}{K_m}$$

or

$$\frac{V}{[S]} = -\frac{1}{K_m}V + \frac{V_{max}}{K_m} \qquad (25)$$

Thus, a plot of $\frac{V}{[S]}$ versus V is linear with a *slope of* $-\frac{1}{K_m}$ and an intercept, of $\frac{V_{max}}{K_m}$ on the $\frac{V}{[S]}$-axis.

When $\frac{V}{[S]}=0$, the intercept on the V-axis, is V_{max}, (Figure 6.3).

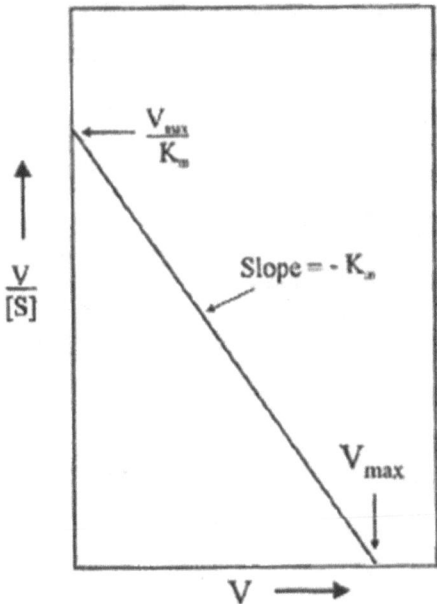

Figure 5.4: *The Eadie-Hofstee plot*

5.7 STEADY STATE KINETICS

5.7.1 Briggs-Haldane Hypothesis

Briggs and Haldane derived a more general expression from application of the steady-state approach for the derivation of equations describing more complex kinetic processes. In the steady-state, the net rate of change of the concentrations of the intermediates are taken as zero, that is, their formation and breakdown are considered dynamically balanced. Furthermore, the concentration of any intermediate is also assumed to be small which for a very a reactive complex such as ES is probably true.

Thus, for the Michaelis-Menten Mechanism

$$E + S \underset{k_{-1}}{\overset{k_1}{\rightleftharpoons}} ES \xrightarrow{k_2} E + P$$

Rate of complex formation = $K_1 \cdot [E] \cdot [S]$,
Rate of complex dissociation = $K_{-1} \cdot [ES]$,
Rate of complex breakdown = $K_2 \cdot [ES]$ and

$$\frac{d[ES]}{dt} = k_1[E][S] - k_{-1}[ES] - k_2[ES]. \qquad (26)$$

Under steady-state conditions,

$$\frac{d[ES]}{dt} = 0.$$

Thus,

$$K_1[E][S] = k_{-1}[ES] + k_2[ES] \qquad (27)$$

Rate of complex formation = Rate of complex dissociation/breakdown.

As before,
$$[E] = [E_0] - [ES],$$

and
$$[S] = [S_0].$$

Therefore,
$$k_1 S_0 (E_0 - ES) = ES \cdot (k_{-1} + k_2)$$

and
$$(E_0 - ES)S_0 = \frac{ES(k_{-1} + k_2)}{k_1} \qquad (28)$$

If the combination of rate constants $\frac{(k_{-1} + k_2)}{k_1}$ is represented as K_M, the rearrangement of equation (28) gives

$$[ES] = \frac{[E_0][S_0]}{S_0 + K_M}$$

But, since $V = k_2 [ES]$

$$V = \frac{k_2 E_0 S_0}{S_0 + K_M} = \frac{V_{max} S_0}{S_0 + K_M} \qquad (29)$$

Equation (29) is the **Briggs-Haldane Equation.** It is identical in form to the Michaelis-Menten equation but is more rigorously derived and more general.

5.8 CASES WHERE INTERMEDIATES OCCURING AFTER [ES]

The M-M equation still applies, although K_m and k_{cat} are combinations of various rate and equilibrium constants. K_m is always less or equal to K_s

Consider the reaction:

$$E + S \xrightleftharpoons{K_s} ES \xrightleftharpoons{k_2} ES' \xrightleftharpoons{k_3} ES'' \xrightleftharpoons[slow]{k_4} EP$$

This involves several intermediates and the final catalytic step is slow. When

$$[ES'] = k_2[ES]; [ES''] = k_3[ES']$$

ES', ES'' are intermediates, EP, final product, k_1, k_2 and k_3 are rate constants.

$$K_m = \frac{K_s}{1 + k_2 + k_3} \qquad (30)$$

and

$$k_{cat} = \frac{k_4 k_2 k_3}{(1 + k_2 + k_2 k_3)}. \qquad (31)$$

For instance, the chymotrypsin-catalysed hydrolysis of esters and amides proceeds through intermediates acylenzyme, as given below:

$$E + S \xrightleftharpoons{K_s} ES \xrightarrow{k_2} EA \xrightarrow{k_3} EP_2$$
$$\phantom{E + S \xrightleftharpoons{K_s} ES \xrightarrow{k_2}} P_1$$

K_s is the dissociation constant of the acylenzyme complex, k_2 and k_3 are rate constants of the acyl intermediates where EA is an 'acylenzyme' intermediate.

ESSENTIALS OF ENZYMOLOGY

Applying steady state assumption to [EA]; it can be shown that:

$$V = [E_0][S] \cdot \left\{ \frac{k_2 k_3 / (k_2 + k_3)}{K_S k_3 / (k_2 + k_3) + [S]} \right\} \qquad (32)$$

Accordingly, cf M-M equation,

$$K_m = K_s \cdot \frac{k_3}{k_2 + k_3}$$

and

$$k_{cat} = \frac{k_2 k_3}{k_2 + k_3}$$

or

$$\frac{1}{k_{cat}} = \frac{1}{k_2} + \frac{1}{k_3}$$

5.9 REVERSIBLE REACTION

All chemical reactions are to some degree reversible. Many enzyme catalyzed reactions can function in either direction within the cell.

Consider the chemical reaction:

$$S \rightleftharpoons P$$

For an enzyme catalysed reaction:

$$E + S \underset{k_{-1}}{\overset{k_1}{\rightleftharpoons}} ES/ES' \underset{k_{-2}}{\overset{k_2}{\rightleftharpoons}} E + P$$

Rate of forward reaction:

$$V_f = k_1 [E][S]$$

Rate of reverse (back) reaction is

$$V_r = k_{-1} [ES]$$

At equilibrium, $V_f = V_r$

$$\frac{[ES]}{[E]} = \frac{k_1 [S]}{k_{-1}}. \qquad (33)$$

In the breakdown of ES to Product:

$$ES \leftrightarrows E + P.$$

Similarly,

$$k_2[ES] = K_{-2}[E][P]$$

$$\frac{[ES]}{[E]} = \frac{k_{-2}[P]}{k_2}. \qquad (34)$$

Combine equations (33) and (34)

$$\frac{k_1[S]}{k_{-1}} = \frac{k_{-2}[P]}{k_2}.$$

At equilibrium,

$$K_{eq} = \frac{[P]}{[S]} = \frac{k_1}{k_{-1}} \times \frac{k_2}{k_{-2}} \qquad (35)$$

Equation (35) shows the relationship between kinetic constant and equilibrium constant for a reversible reaction.

On applying the Michaelis-Menten (M-M) equation, the Forward reaction at fixed $[E_0]$ is given by

$$V_f = \frac{V_{max}^S [S_0]}{[S_0] + K_m^S} \qquad (36)$$

where v_f = initial velocity in the forward reaction and V_{max}^S = maximum velocity

$$K_m^S = \frac{k_{-1} + k_2}{k_1}.$$

Similarly the M-M equation for the Reverse (Back)-Reaction

$$V_r = \frac{V_{max}^P \cdot [P_0]}{[P_0] + K_m^P}$$

Where, V_r = initial velocity of the reverse reaction; V_{max}^P = maximum velocity, then

$$K_m^P = \frac{k_{-1} + k_2}{k_{-2}}.$$

Substituting for kinetic equilibrium equation (6.27) above

$$K_{eq} = \frac{k_1 k_2}{k_{-1} \cdot k_{-2}} = \frac{V_{max}^S K_m^P}{V_{max}^P \cdot K_m^S} \qquad (37)$$

Equation (37) is referred to as **Haldane Relation.** This shows the relationship between kinetic constant and equilibrium constant for a reversible reaction.

5.10 MEASUREMENT OF RATE CONSTANTS

The catalytic reaction is divided into two steps: namely

(i) the formation of enzyme-substrate complex and
(ii) the breakdown of the complex to form products and regeneration of the enzyme (Scheme 1)

$$E + S \underset{}{\overset{K_S}{\rightleftharpoons}} ES \xrightarrow{k_{cat}} E + P$$

Scheme 1

The first step is rapid and reversible and there is no chemical change. Thus, E, S, and ES equilibrate very rapidly. The second step is a chemical process, at which the enzyme-substrate complex, ES breaks down to product, P with the regeneration of the enzyme. The instantaneous velocity at any time depends on the concentration of ES.

$$V = k_{cat} \cdot ES$$

k_{cat} is called the *catalytic rate constant.* It is a first order rate constant. Also, it corresponds to the *turnover number* of the enzyme because it represents the maximum number of substrate molecules converted to products per active site per unit time, or the number of times the enzyme "turns over" per unit time. For complex reactions, k_{cat} is a function of all the first order rate constant and cannot be assigned to any particular process.

The k_{cat} value may be the combination of the rate constants for several steps. The measurement of rate of approach to the steady state enables one to detect transient intermediates, and also to observe the individual rate constants. The value of k_{cat} lie between 1 and 10^7 sec^{-1}. Therefore measurements must be made in the time range of $1 - 10^7$ sec^{-1}. This requires techniques for rapidly mixing and then observing the enzyme and substrate. Two types of techniques have been developed. The first is *Rapid-mixing,* whereby two solutions can be mixed in a fraction of millisecond, since majority of enzyme turnover numbers are less than 1000 sec^{-1}. The second is *Relaxation kinetics*, in which the time barrier due to mixing is overcome by using pre-mixed solutions.

5.11 RAPID-MIXING AND QUENCHING TECHNIQUES

These comprise two methods: Continuous-flow method and Stopped-flow method. Hatridge and Roughton introduced the continuous flow method to solution kinetics for the pioneering work on studies of ligand binding to haemoglobin. The principle of the method is illustrated in Figure 5.5.

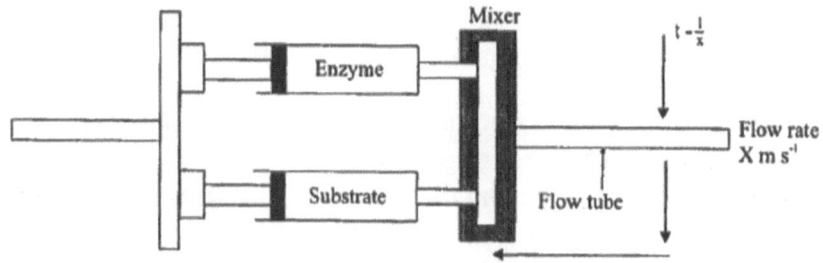

Figure 5.5: Continuous flow apparatus

(i) Continuous Flow Method

Two syringes are connected by a mixing chamber to a flow tube. One syringe is filled with the enzyme, the other with substrate, and the two are compressed at a constant rate. The two solutions mix thoroughly in the mixing chamber, then passes down the flow tube and 'age'. At a constant flow, the age of the solution is linearly proportional to the distance down the flow tube and the flow rate. The flow rate of the liquid must be kept above a critical velocity in order to ensure 'turbulent flow'; otherwise the flow may be laminar. This places an upper limit on the apparatus for a particular length of tube.

(ii) Stopped Flow Method

This was devised by Roughton in 1934 and later improved upon by Chance. The principle is illustrated in Figure 5.6.

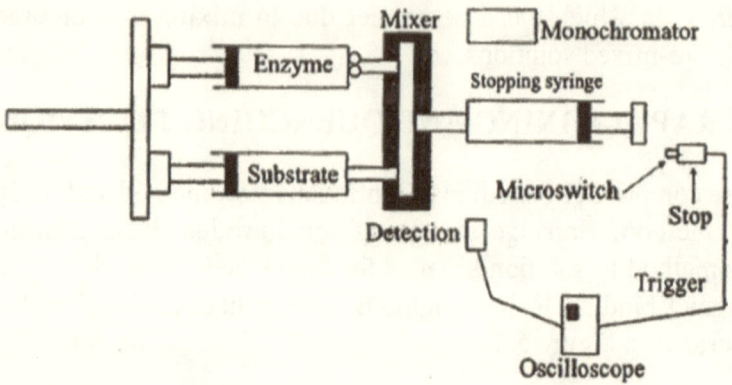

Figure 5.6: Stopped-flow apparatus

The apparatus is a slight modification of that for the Continuous flow method. The two driving syringes are compressed to expel about 50-200 µl from each syringe and then mechanically stopped.

Observation points are located along the tube adjoining the mixing chamber. Suppose the flow rate is 10 ms^{-1} during the period of compression, and the observation point is 1 cm after the mixing chamber, the detector sees a solution during this continuous flow period and the solution is 1 ms old. The age of the solution at the initial observation is known as the "dead time" of the apparatus. It has a dead time as low as 0.5ms., and so enables observation to be extended to several minutes. However, it requires a rapid detection and recording system. The continuous-flow system requires very large reaction volumes and readings may be taken only up to about 100ms or so, due to the impracticalities of using longer observation tubes.

This method is a routine laboratory tool as compared to the continuous flow method. The advantage of this technique is that it requires only 100 – 400 µl of solution or less for complete time course of a reaction.

(iii) Quenching Techniques

These arise from the modifications of the methods mentioned above which eliminate the use of a photo multiplier or other detector in the flow systems. These are called rapid quenching techniques, because the solutions may be quenched by the addition of an acid, for example, trichloroacetic acid and then the reaction products directly analysed by chromatographic or other techniques. The two important types of these techniques are (a) quenched - flow technique and (b) the pulsed-quenched flow technique.

In case of quenched-flow method, the end of the observation tube of a continuous flow apparatus (see Figure 6.4) is submerged in a beaker of acid. In a typical apparatus, third syringe is added which mixes the quenching acid with the reagent solutions via a second mixing chamber. The dead time of only 4 or 5ms is obtainable in such apparatus.

For the pulsed -quenched flow method, the apparatus and procedure are similar to that of the stopped-flow. The enzyme and substrate are first mixed and driven into an incubation tube by a plunger actuated by compressed air, and after the desired time interval, 150ms or greater, a second plunger is actuated which drives the incubated mixture with a pulse of distilled water into a second mixer where it is quenched.

5.12 RELAXATION METHODS

These methods involve the measurement of rate constant of reactions which have attained an equilibrium state. Thus, the rate constant is measured for an equilibrium mixture of the reagents already incubated together. Of note, chemical equilibrium are usually affected by one or more of the following parameters: pressure, temperature and electric field. Generally, the system is perturbed from its equilibrium position and its rate of relaxation to a new equilibrium is measured. This principle has been applied in the temperature jump technique, which is the most common relaxation method for the measurement of rate constant in enzymic reaction.

In this method, the solution is incubated in an absorbance or fluorescence cell and its temperature is raised through $5 - 10°$ in less than a microsecond by the discharge of a capacitor or by an infra-red laser. Due to the enthalpy change, the equilibrium position will change. This is represented by the equation, called the Van't Hoff equation,

$$\Delta H = RT^2 \frac{d \ln K_{eq}}{dT}.$$

Hence,

$$\frac{d \ln K_{eq}}{dT} = \frac{\Delta H}{RT^2}$$

Where, H is the Enthalpy; R, the gas constant; K_{eq}, the equilibrium constant and T, the absolute temperature.

The system will proceed to its new equilibrium position via a series of relaxation times, τ, which is the reciprocal of the rate constant.

CHAPTER SIX

Enzyme Kinetics II

6.0 MULTISUBSTRATE ENZYME CATALYSED REACTIONS

Most biochemical reactions involve at least two substrates: thus, it is necessary to consider the kinetics of such reactions. This is an extremely complex topic but for simplicity we will restrict discussion on the specific examples which involve two-substrates and two products (Bi-Bi-Reaction). Such reactions can be classified into two mechanistic classes which are termed, Sequential and Ping-Pong (Non-sequential).

Nomenclature of Multisubstrate Reactions

Cleland had designated multisubstrate enzyme catalysed reactions according to (a) No of substrates and products, and (b) the reaction mechanism. Essentially, the reactancy is equal to the number of kinetically significant substrates or products. It is designated by the syllables: UNI, BI, TER, QUAD. Examples of these reactions are illustrated below:

(a) $A \to P$ — Uni : Uni
(b) $A \to P + Q$ — Uni : Bi
(c) $A + B \to P$ — Bi : Uni
(d) $A + B \to P + Q$ — Bi : Bi
(e) $A + B + C \to P + Q$ — Ter : Bi

6.1 SEQUENTIAL MECHANISM

In this case, both substrates bind to the enzyme to form a ternary complex before the products are formed and released. This can be illustrated by the following reaction sequence:

$$E + S_1 + S_2 \longleftrightarrow ES_1S_2 \longleftrightarrow E + P_1 + P_2$$

Depending on the order of addition of the substrates, this class can be subdivided into reaction mechanisms, in which substrates associate and products dissociate either at Random or in an Ordered fashion. These are referred to as *random sequential* and *ordered sequential* respectively.

(i) Random Sequential

The ternary complex, $ES_1 S_2$ is formed via either the binary complexes ES_1 or S_2 as intermediates, and the enzyme therefore possesses distinct sites for both substrates. The random mechanism can be represented as follows:

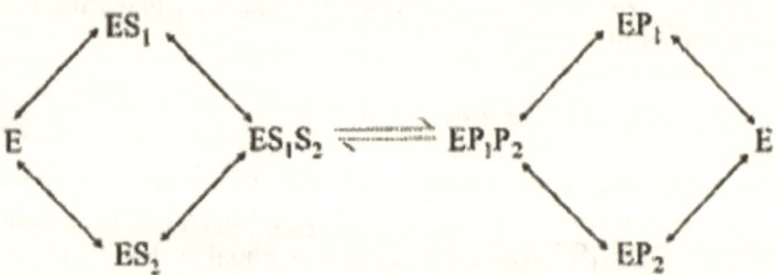

S_1 - EOH, S_2 = ATP: P_1 = R.PO$_4$ P_2 - ADP.

Examples of enzymes which exhibit this mode of reaction mechanism include:

(a) Creatine phosphokinase (R = Creatine)
(b) Pyruvate kinase (R = Pyruvate)
(c) Hexo kinase (R = Glucose)

(ii) Ordered Sequential

In an Ordered sequential reaction, the two substrates add in a *compulsory order* to the enzyme:

$$E + S_1 \longleftrightarrow ES_1 \xleftrightarrow{S_2} ES_1S_2 \longleftrightarrow EP_1P_2 \longleftrightarrow EP_2 \longleftrightarrow EP_1P_2$$

This mechanism is often associated with many enzymes exhibiting coenzyme requirements; for example; lactate dehydrogenase, alcohol dehydrogenase. The coenzyme can be envisaged to bind first to a specific, complementary site on the enzyme so as to provide a reactive coenzyme for the 2nd substrate.

Example: Alcohol dehydrogenase (Horse – Liver) which catalyses the oxidation of ethanol to acetaldehyde.

$$C_2H_5OH \xleftrightarrow{ALDH} CH_3CHO$$

This has been found to exhibit a modified version of this mechanism known as *Theorell-Chance mechanism.*

6.2 NON-SEQUENTIAL MECHANISM (*Ping-pong*)

This is an ordered reaction in which the enzyme oscillates between the different substrates. It is made up of two partial reactions as shown below:

$$E + S_1 \longrightarrow ES_1 \longrightarrow EP_1 \longrightarrow \begin{array}{c} E^1 + S_2 \\ + \\ P_1 \end{array} \quad (i)$$

$$E^1S_2 \longleftrightarrow E^1P_2 \longleftrightarrow E^1 + P_2 \quad (ii)$$

where S_1 = RCO_2R; S_2 = H_2O; E^1 = E-O-CO-R; P_1 = ROH and P_2 = $R.CO_2H$.

Examples of enzymes which exhibit this mechanism include:

(a) hydrolytic enzymes where the second acceptor is water,
(b) transaminases: S_1 = L-aspartate, S_2 = oxoglutarate
                                  P_2 = oxaloacetate P_1 = glutamate
                                  $E' = (E\text{-}MH_2)$

6.3 KINETICS OF BISUBSTRATE REACTIONS

6.3.1 General Consideration

The development of kinetic theory of bisubstrate reaction has been due mainly to the work of Alberty and his co-workers, Dalziel, Cleland, Hanes and Wong. The experimental facts on which this theory is based are quite analogous to those of one-substrate reactions: the variation of the initial velocity as a function of the concentration of one of the two substrates (e.g. [A] then called the variable substrate) is given by a **Michaelis-Menten equation.**

$$V_0 = \frac{V_{max}[A]}{K_A + [A]} \quad (6.1)$$

$$\frac{1}{V_0} = K_A \cdot \frac{1}{[A]} + \frac{1}{V_{max}} \quad (6.2)$$

Provided that

(i) the same restrictions are observed especially with respect to the absence of products and
(ii) that the second substrate, (here [B], the fixed substrate is held constant at a concentration [B] >> [E_0].

If a similar set of measurements is then carried out at different concentrations $[B]_2$ >> [E_0], again the variation of the initial velocity as a function of [A] follows the Michaeli-Menten equation, but now it usually yields a different value for the two kinetic parameters V and

K_A; they are, therefore functions of the concentration of [B] as well. In general, the pattern of the reciprocal plots is that of two families of straight lines as shown in Figure 6.1.

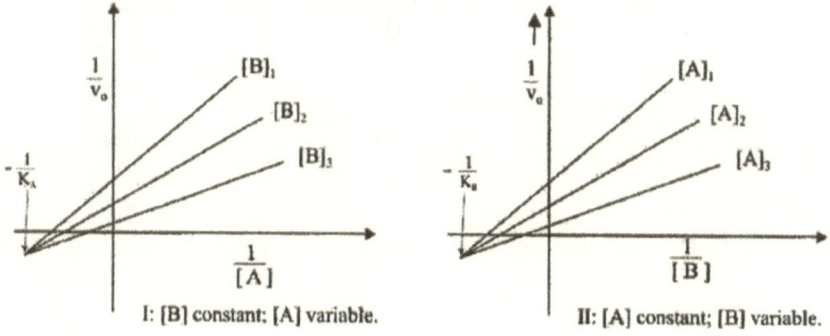

I: [B] constant; [A] variable.   II: [A] constant; [B] variable.

Figure 6.1: *Double reciprocal plots for bisubstrate reactions*

For the two-substrate reaction, the kinetic equation requires a total of four kinetic parameters, V, K_m^A, K_m^B and $\overline{K}_m$; $K_{\overline{m}}$. This set is both necessary and sufficient for a unique description of the kinetics. In case of one substrate reaction, only two parameters are required; V; K_M.

6.4 DERIVATION OF RATE EQUATION FOR TWO-SUBSTRATE REACTION

Consider the reaction:

$$E + A \xrightleftharpoons{K_A} EA + B$$
$$\searrow K_m^B$$
$$EAB \longrightarrow ECD \longrightarrow E + C + D$$
$$\nearrow K_m^A$$
$$E + B \xrightleftharpoons{K_B} EB + A$$

At rapid equilibrium condition; the simple dissociation constants are as follows:

$$K_A = \frac{[E][A]}{[EA]}; \qquad K_B = \frac{[E][B]}{[EB]} \qquad (6.3)$$

$$K_M^A = \frac{[E][A]}{[EA]}; \qquad K_M^B \cdot \frac{[EA][B]}{[EAB]} \qquad (6.4)$$

The rate of product formation is directly proportional to [EAB], thus

$$V_0 = K_2[EAB].$$

By the Conservation law,

$$E_0 = [E] + [EA] + [EB] + [EAB] \qquad (6.5)$$

Since there are four equations to which to convert the three unknowns [EA], [EB], [EAB], one equation is redundant (the four constants are interrelated, thus:

$$K_A K_M^B = K_B K_M^A \qquad (6.6)$$

Hence the rate equation is given by

$$V_0 = \frac{V_{max}}{1 + K_M^A/[A] + K_M^B/[B] + K_A \cdot K_M^B/[A][B]} \qquad (6.7)$$

Equation (1) is the most general rate equation for two-substrate kinetics which describes adequately a number of enzyme-catalysed reactions.

This equation corresponds to an ordered two-substrate reactions.

6.5 STEADY STATE KINETICS FOR MULTI-SUBSTRATE REACTIONS

Many two-substrates enzyme catalysed reactions obey the Michaelis-Menten equation in respect to one substrate at constant concentrations of the other substrate. This applies both to the reaction catalysed by enzymes with just one binding site per substrate and by those with several binding sites per substrate provided there is no interaction between the binding sites. For such reactions, Alberty (1953) derived the general equations as follows:

$$AX + B \rightleftharpoons BX + A.$$

$$V_0 = \frac{V_{max}[AX_0][B_0]}{K_m^B[AX_0] + K_m^{AX}[B_0] + [AX_0][B_0] + K_1^{AX} \cdot K_m^B} \quad (6.8)$$

where V_{max} maximum velocity when AX and B are both saturating, K_S^{AX} = Concentration of AX which gives $\frac{1}{2} V_{max}$ when B is saturating, K_m^B = Concentration of B which gives $\frac{1}{2} V_{max}$ when AX is saturating and K_S^{AX} = dissociating constant for the enzyme substrate complex, EAX. The assumption that the total enzyme concentration is constant and much smaller than the concentration of the two substrates.

At very large $[B_0]$, the general equation simplifies to:

$$V_0 = \frac{V_{max}}{1 + K_m^{AX}/[AX_0]} = \frac{V_{max}[AX_0]}{AX_0 + K_m^{AX}} \quad (6.9)$$

Similarly, at very large $[AX_0]$

$$V_0 = \frac{V_{max}}{1 + K_m^B/[B_0]} = \frac{V_{max}[B_0]}{[B_0] + K_m^B} \quad (6.10)$$

Similar rate equations for the bisubstrate reactions have been developed by other biochemists, Cleland (1963) and Bloomfield (1963). These workers have employed different symbolics.

Alberty (1956):

$$\frac{V}{V_0} = 1 + \frac{K_A}{A} + \frac{K_B}{B} + \frac{K_{AB}}{AB} \qquad (6.11)$$

Bloomfield *et al.* (1963):

$$\frac{V_{AB}}{V_0} = 1 + \frac{K_{AB}}{K_B}\frac{1}{A} + \frac{K_{AB}}{K_A}\cdot\frac{1}{B} + \frac{K_{AB}}{AB} \qquad (6.12)$$

Cleland (1963):

$$\frac{V}{V_0} = 1 + \frac{K_a}{A} + \frac{K_b}{B} + \frac{K_{ia}K_b}{AB}. \qquad (6.13)$$

Table: Comparison of different symbolisms of bisubtrate kinetics

Enzyme Commission	Meaning	Alberty	Bloomfield *et al.*	Cleland
K_m^A	Limiting Michaelis constant for A	k_a	$\dfrac{K_{AB}}{K_B}$	K_a
K_m^B	Limiting Michaelis constant for B	K_B	$\dfrac{K_{AB}}{K_A}$	K_b
K_a	Dissociating constant for A	$\dfrac{K_{AB}}{K_B}$	V_{AB}	K_{ia}
V	Limiting maximum velocity	V_f	V_{AB}	V_1
None	Turnover number	$\dfrac{V_1}{E_0}$	$\dfrac{V_{AB}}{E_0}$	$\dfrac{V_1}{E_0}$

6.6 NON-LINEAR KINETICS

Allosteric enzymes exhibit sigmoid kinetics curves rather than hyperbola in plots of initial velocity against substrate concentration (Figure 6.2). Generally, they play a regulatory role in intermediate metabolism. Thus, the region in which velocity is most sensitive to substrate concentration is moved out to the physiological concentration range. The particular conditions found to yield regulatory behaviour commonly include:

(i) the presence of an 'effector' molecule which may be an activator or an inhibitor of the enzyme activity
(ii) metabolites that may be or may not be the substrate of the enzyme

The sigmoid behaviour may be exhibited under similar or different conditions namely:

(i) Errors in substrate concentration.
(ii) Presence of mixed enzymes.
(iii) Existence of non-linear two-substrate mechanisms.
(iv) Presence of multiple interacting substrate sites.
(v) Separate substrate and effector subunits.
(vi) Multiple identical subunits with non-co-operative binding.

The concept of 'Allosterism' emanated from the idea that substrate molecules and molecules of regulatory metabolites occupy different locations on the enzyme as suggested by the chemical dissimilarity of specific substrates and specific effectors in many cases. Hence, the term *allosteric effects.*

Examples of allosteric enzymes are phosphofructokinase, (PFK); Aspartate transcarbomylase.

Allosteric (*allo = other*) interactions describe those interactions between ligands bound to the protein at some distance from one another. These can be either **Homotropic** – those between **LIKE** *molecules* or **Heterotropic** – those between **UNLIKE** *molecules.*

6.6.1 Features of Allostery

(i) Lack of chemical resemblance between substrate and the effector.
(ii) Sigmoid shape (kinetic behaviour)
(iii) Changes in protein conformation.
(iv) Oligomeric nature of the protein
(v) Exhibition of positive or negative co-operativity.

6.6.2 Comparison of Allosteric Enzymes Activity

Koshland, Nemethyl and Filmer have proposed the useful parameter, for comparing activity of control enzymes. This is given by the "Cooperativity factor", R_S where,

$$R_S = \frac{\text{Substrate (or ligand) concentration at 0.9 saturation level}}{\text{Substrate (or ligand) concentration at 0.1 saturation level}}$$

for an enzyme that follow Michaelis-Menten kinetics, $R_S = 81$.

For an enzymes that exhibit Sigmoid kinetics, $R_S < 81$.

Positive cooperativity is exhibited when $R_S > 81$ that is, the binding of the substrate becomes easy as the enzyme becomes more and more saturated.

Negative Cooperativity ($R_S < 81$) is exhibited when the binding of the substrate get progressively more difficult as the enzyme becomes saturated.

6.7 LIGAND-BINDING TO ALLOSTERIC PROTEIN

The classical allosteric protein which has been studied extensively is Haemoglobin. If we consider, the oxygen – binding phenomenon of this protein, the following features are exhibited clearly:

(i) The shape of the oxygen dissociation curve of haemoglobin is sigmoidal.

(ii) This shows that the binding of oxygen to haemoglobin is of the cooperative nature.
(iii) The affinity of haemoglobin for oxygen depends on pH. The CO_2 molecule also affects the oxygen binding characteristics of haemoglobin.

The oxygen affinity of haemoglobin is further regulated by organic phosphates such as diphosphoglycerate. These regulatory molecules profoundly alter the oxygen binding properties of haemoglobin, although, they are bound to sites on the protein that are far from the hemes.

The saturation, $\bar{Y}$ is defined as the fractional occupancy of the oxygen – binding sites. The value of $\bar{Y}$ can range from 0 (all sites filled) to 1.0. The plot of $\bar{Y}$ versus pO_2 the partial pressure of oxygen is called an ***oxygen dissociation curve.***

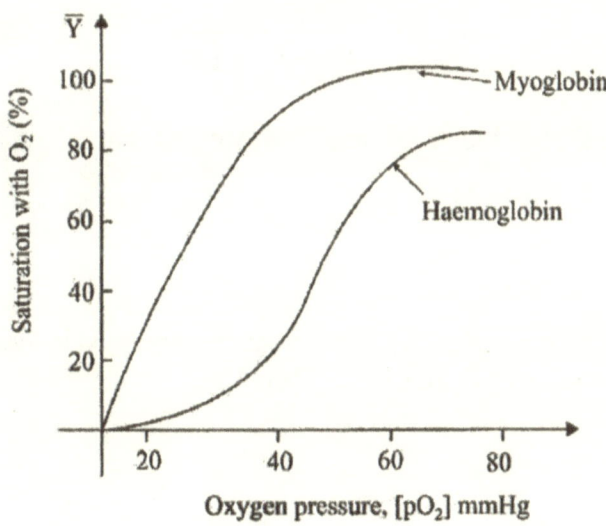

Figure 6.2: Oxygen dissociation curve of Myoglobin and Haemoglobin

6.8 KINETICS OF LIGAND-BINDING TO HEMOPROTEINS [MYOGLOBIN & HAEMOGLOBIN]

Consider myoglobin, a monomeric protein which binds one molecule of oxygen.

(i) Myoglobin

$$MbO_2 = Mb + O_2$$

$$K_b = \frac{[Mb][O_2]}{[MbO_2]} \qquad (6.14)$$

where $[MbO_2]$ is the concentration of oxymyoglobin (moles/litre) and $[O_2]$ the concentration of uncombined O_2.

$$\text{Fractional saturation, } \bar{Y} = \frac{[MbO_2]}{[MbO_2] + [Mb]} \qquad (6.15)$$

Substituting equation (6.14) into (6.15) we find that

$$\bar{Y} = \frac{[O_2]}{[O_2] + K_b} \qquad (6.16)$$

Since oxygen is a gas, concentration can be expressed in terms of pO_2 (partial pressure of O_2 in torrs.). Therefore,

$$\bar{Y} = \frac{pO_2}{pO_2 + p_{50}}. \qquad (6.17)$$

Equation (6.17) plot is a hyperbola.

The oxygen dissociation curve calculated from equation (6.17) taking pO_2 to be 1 torr closely matches the experimental data. The binding relationship that could be derived from equation (6.17) is given as:

$$\frac{\bar{Y}}{1-\bar{Y}} = \frac{pO_2}{P_{50}} \qquad (6.18)$$

A plot of log $\frac{\bar{Y}}{1-\bar{Y}}$ versus log PO_2 yields a straight line with a slope 1.

This representation is called a **Hill plot** and its slope (n) is called the **Hill coefficient.** (See Figure 6.3)

(ii) Haemoglobin (Tetrameric Protein)

$$Hb + nO_2 = Hb(O_2)n$$

where n is the number of binding sites per Hb molecule. The Binding constant is given by

$$K_b = \frac{[Hb(O_2)n]}{[Hb]+[Hb(O_2)n]} \qquad (6.19)$$

where pO_2 = partial pressure of O_2. Therefore

$$[Hb(O_2)n] = K_b \times pO_2^n \, [Hb]$$

Fractional Saturation, $\bar{Y} = \frac{[Hb(O_2)n]}{[Hb] + [Hb(O_2)n]} \qquad (6.20)$

Substituting for $[Hb(O_2)n]$ from equation (6.19) reduces equation (6.20) to

$$\bar{Y} = \frac{K_b \cdot [pO_2]^n \cdot [Hb]}{[Hb] + K_b[pO_2]^n \cdot [Hb]} \qquad (6.21)$$

and so

$$\bar{Y} = \frac{K_b \cdot [pO_2]^n}{1 + K_b \cdot [pO_2]^n} \qquad (6.22)$$

If n = 1, that is only one O_2 binding site per protein subunit, we find

$$\bar{Y} = \frac{K_b \cdot [pO_2]}{1 + K_b \cdot [pO_2]^n}$$

But

$$\frac{[Hb(O_2)n]}{[Hb]} = K_b[pO_2]^n \qquad (6.23),$$

then

$$\frac{\bar{Y}}{1-\bar{Y}} = Kb[pO_2]^n. \qquad (6.24)$$

Taking the log of both sides:

$$\log \frac{\bar{Y}}{1-\bar{Y}} = \log K_b + n \log pO_2 \qquad (6.25).$$

The Hill plot for the binding of oxygen to haemoglobin is depicted in Figure 6.3. The Hill's coefficient is 2.8.

6.9 QUANTITATIVE ANALYSIS OF COOPERATIVITY

If an enzyme containing n binding constants and all n are occupied simultaneously with a dissociation constant K. This can be expressed as follows

$$E + nS \xrightleftharpoons{K} ES_n \qquad (6.26)$$

Thus,

$$K = \frac{[E][S]^n}{[ES]_n} \qquad (6.27)$$

The degree of saturation, $\overline{Y}$ is given by

$$\overline{Y} = \frac{ES_n}{[E_0]} \qquad (6.28)$$

and
$$1 - \overline{Y} = \frac{[E]}{[E_0]} \qquad (6.29)$$

Equations (6.27) and (6.29) may be manipulated to give

$$\log\left[\frac{\overline{Y}}{[1-\overline{Y}]}\right] = n \log [S] - \log K \qquad (6.30)$$

This is similar to *Hill plot,* equation (6.25), which describes satisfactorily the binding of ligands to allosteric proteins in region of 50% saturation, (10 - 90%). Outside this region, the experimental curve deviates from the straight line.

The value of n found from the slope of graphical plot, (Figure 6.3) in the region of 50% saturation is known as the *Hill constant.* It is a measure of cooperativity. The higher the n is the higher the cooperativity. At the upper limit, n is equal to the number of binding sites. If n = 1, there is no cooperativity. If n>1 there is positive cooperativity, if n<1 there is negative cooperativity.

6.10 KINETICS OF LIGAND-BINDING TO AN ALLOSTERIC ENZYME MOLECULE

In case of enzyme catalysed reaction, in which the velocity of the reaction is determined by the concentration of E – S complex, a fraction saturating of unity is equivalent to the maximum velocity, V_{max}. Thus, a *Hill Plot* consists of a plot of $\log \frac{v_0}{V_{max} - v_0}$ against log S where v_0 = initial velocity at a given substrate concentration, S.

Consider the enzyme, E and the ligand, say A.

$$E + nA \xrightleftharpoons{k_a} [EA]_n \xrightleftharpoons{k_2} E + nX$$

The Binding Constant k_a is given by

$$k_a = \frac{[EA]_n}{[E].[nA]} \qquad (6.31)$$

Note that,

$$K_a = \frac{1}{k_s}.$$

$$E_0 = E + [EA]_n \qquad (6.32)$$

Where, E_0 = (Total Enzyme) and E = (Free enzyme).

But

$$V_{max} = k_2[EA]_n \qquad (6.33)$$

Also,

$$v_0 = k_2 E_0 \qquad (6.34)$$

Assuming v_0 is proportional to [EA], concentration of enzyme bound substrate.

At Steady state conditions, where $[A] \ggg [E_0]$; $[A] = [A_0]$

$$\frac{v_0}{V_{max}} = \frac{[EA]}{[E_0]} = \bar{Y}$$

Hence,

$$\frac{\overline{Y}}{1-\overline{Y}} = \frac{V_o}{V_{max} - V_o}$$

Thus, the plot of $\log\left(\dfrac{V_o}{V_{max} - V_o}\right)$ against log [A] gives the slope, Hill coefficient, (h), which is equal to the number of binding sites, (n).

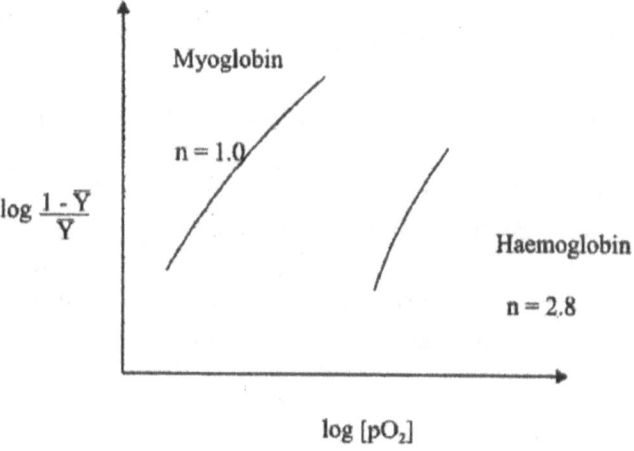

Figure 6.3: *Hill plots for the binding of Oxygen to Myogblobin and Haemoglobin*

CHAPTER SEVEN

Enzyme Kinetic III

7.0 ENZYME INHIBITION

The rate of an enzyme catalysed reaction can be altered in a specific manner by compounds other than the substrates. Activators increase the rate whilst the inhibitors are substances which tend to decrease the rate of an enzyme catalysed reaction. Some act as substrate or co-factor, and some may combine directly with an enzyme. There are two main groups of inhibitors – *reversible inhibitors* and *irreversible inhibitors*. Some important inhibitors of interest to the biochemist are listed in Table 7.1.

Table 7.1: *Some Important Inhibitors*

Compound	Postulated mode of Action	Reaction Enzyme affected
Organophosphorus / compounds $R_1O\diagdown\underset{R_2O\diagup}{P}\underset{X}{\diagup O}$	Covalent bond to serine-OH	Trypsin, choline-sterase phospho-glucomutase etc.
Organic mercurials X-Hg-Ar	Covalent mercaptide bond to cysteine-SH = protein-S-Hg Ar reversed by addition of R'SH in excess	Large number of enzymes.

Heavy metals; Ag^+, Hg^+	Formation of covalent metal salts; protein-SK, $-CO_2^-$; histidine	Large number of enzymes, e.g. fructose furanosidate: Ag^+-histidine.
Metal-complexing; CN^-, S^-, N^{-3} agents: (low concentrations)	Formation of complex with metallo- enzymes, especially metalloporphyrins and copper enzymes	cytochrome oxidase, catalase, urate oxidase etc.
: -CO -	Same as above	Cytochrome oxidase polyphenol oxidase
: CN^-, S^-, N_3^-, F^-	Formation of complex with metalloenzymes as above or removal of metals (Cu, Fe, Mo, Zn, Hg, etc.) from enzymes	Large number of metalloenzymes
Derivatives of iodoacetate ICH_2COR	Formation of S-alkyl derivatives of cysteine = protein -s- CH_2COR	Large number of enzymes, e.g. glyceradehyde-β dehydrogenase.
Fluorocitrate $$\begin{array}{c} CHF\ CO_2^- \\ | \\ HO-C-CO_2^- \\ | \\ CH_2CO_2^- \end{array}$$	Competitive inhibitor for citrate	Aconitase, citric acid cycle.
Monoguanidines $$\begin{array}{c} H_2N-CNH(CH_2)_nCH_3 \\ \| \\ NH \end{array}$$	Competitive inhibitor for monoamines	Monoanine oxidase, brain and nerve funtion.
Sulfonamides $RNH-\underset{\underset{O}{\|}}{\overset{\overset{O}{\|}}{S}}-\bigcirc-NH_2$	Competitive inhibitor of p- aminobenzoate	Formation of folic acid and hence all folic acid coenzyme dependent reactions in susceptible organisms.
Folic acid analogs: Aminopterin; amethopterin etc.	Competitive inhibitor of folate	Reduction of folate and dihydrofolate and hence of formation of methionine, thymine, purines.

Pyridine-3-sulfonate	Competitive inhibitor of nicotinic acid	Biosynthesis of nicotinamide coenzymes.
Avidin: (Protein from egg-white)	Binds to Biotin	Inhibits all biotin enzymes.
5-methyl tryptophan	Competitive inbihitor of trytophan	Blocks formation of tryptophan-tRNA acid hence protein synthesis.
Azaserine: $N_2=CH-C(=O)-O-CH_2\,CHCO_2^-$ $\quad\quad\quad\quad\quad\quad\quad\quad\; {}^+NH_3$	Competitive inhibitor of glutamine	Competes with gluramine in $-NH_2$ transfer reactions of purane synthesis.
5-Fluoro-deoxyuridine-5'-P	Competitive inhibitor of uridylate	Competes in thymidylate synthetase and hence blocks DNA synthesis
Puromycin	Competitive with aminoacyl-tRNA	Prevents completion of nascent polypeptide chains in protein synthesis.

These substances provide powerful tools for studying the chemical mechanisms of enzyme action.

Reversible Inhibitors bind to the enzyme in a reversible manner and can be removed by dialysis. They usually form an equilibrium system with an enzyme rapidly to show a definite degree of inhibition, depending on the concentration of enzyme, inhibitor and substrate. *Irreversible* Inhibitors bind irreversibly to the enzyme and cannot be removed from the enzyme, whilst degree of inhibition may increase over this period of time.

7.1 TYPES OF REVERSIBLE INHIBITION

7.1.1 Competitive Inhibition

This inhibition is a classical type of reversible inhibition. For example, malonate (malonic acid) is a competitive inhibitor in the reaction which involves the conversion of succinate to fumarate in the Kreb's cycle. This reaction is catalysed by succinate dehydrogenase enzyme. Malonate bears close resemblance in structure to the substrate, succinate. The inhibition involves no covalent bonds. It is instantaneous rather than progressive.

$$CO_2CH_2CH_2CO_2 \underset{\text{Dehydrogenase}}{\overset{\text{Succinic}}{\rightleftharpoons}} \begin{array}{c} CO_2 \\ | \\ CH \\ \| \\ CH \\ | \\ CO_2 \end{array}$$

Succinate　　　　　　　　　　　　　Fumarate

Conversion of succinate to fumarate

$$\begin{array}{cc} COO^- & COO^- \\ | & | \\ CH_2 & CH_2 \\ | & | \\ COO^- & CH_2 \\ & | \\ & COO^- \end{array}$$

Malonate　　　　Succinate

Kinetics of Competitive Inhibition

Consider the reaction:

$$E + S \xrightleftharpoons[K_{-1}]{K_1} ES \xrightarrow{K_2} E + P$$
$$\updownarrow I$$
$$EI$$

Diagrammatically,

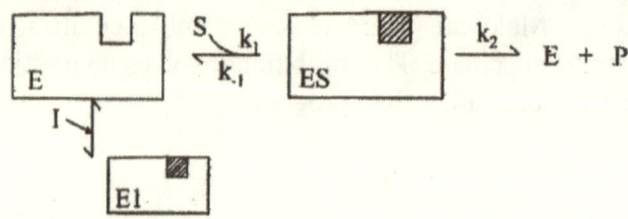

Diagrammatic representation of competitive inhibition at the active site

I = Inhibitor: EI, = Enzyme - Inhibitor Complex, [S], substrate, E, enzyme

$$E + I \rightleftharpoons EI$$

$$K_i = \frac{(E)(I)}{(EI)} \qquad (7.1)$$

At steady state

$$k_1[E][S] = k_{-1} + k_2[ES]$$

$$ES = \frac{[E][S]}{(k_{-1} + k_2)/k_1} \qquad (7.2)$$

If

$$K_m = \frac{k_{-1} + k_2}{k_1}$$

Thus,

$$[ES] = \frac{[E][S]}{K_m} \qquad (7.3)$$

But

$$[E_0] = [E] + [ES] + [EI]$$

$$= [E] + [ES] + \frac{[E][I]}{k_i} \qquad (7.4)$$

$$= [E]\left[1 + \frac{[I]}{k_i}\right] + ES \qquad (7.5)$$

Therefore,

$$[E] = \frac{[E_0] - [ES]}{\left[1 + \frac{[I]}{K_i}\right]}$$

On substituting for (E) in equation (7.3); we find

$$\frac{[E_0] - [ES] \times [S]}{\left[1 + \frac{[I]}{k_i}\right] + [ES]} = K_m \qquad (7.6)$$

$$\frac{[E_0] - [ES]}{[ES]}[S] = K_m\left[1 + \frac{[I]}{k_i}\right]$$

Since

$$V_{max} = k_2[ES]$$

and

$$[ES] = \frac{[E_0]}{1 + \frac{K_m}{[S]}\left(1 + \frac{I}{k_i}\right)} \qquad (7.7)$$

Hence,

$$V_0 = \frac{V_{max}[S_0]}{[S_0] + K_m\left(1 + \frac{[I_0]}{k_i}\right)} \qquad (7.8)$$

Note: From equation (7.8) when compared with the Michaelis-Menten equation:

(a) Km is increased by a factor $1 + \dfrac{[I_0]}{k_i}$

(b) V_{max} is unchanged.

Thus, the inhibitor binds to [E] but not to [ES] complex. It is competitive and the V_{max} for the Lineweaver–Buck plot is unchanged.

7.2 NON-COMPETITIVE INHIBITION

This mode of inhibition has been referred to as "inhibition without affinity" since the inhibitor is not bound at the substrate binding site but at some other binding sites on the enzyme. See Figure 7.3.

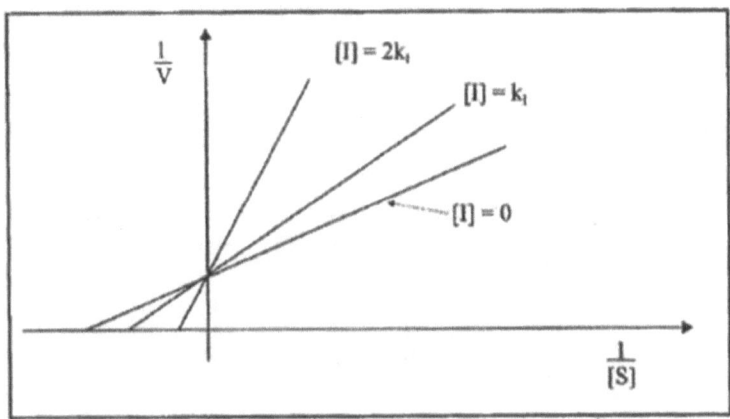

Figure 7.2: *Lineweaver-Burke plot for competitive inhibition*
[I] is the inhibitor concentration

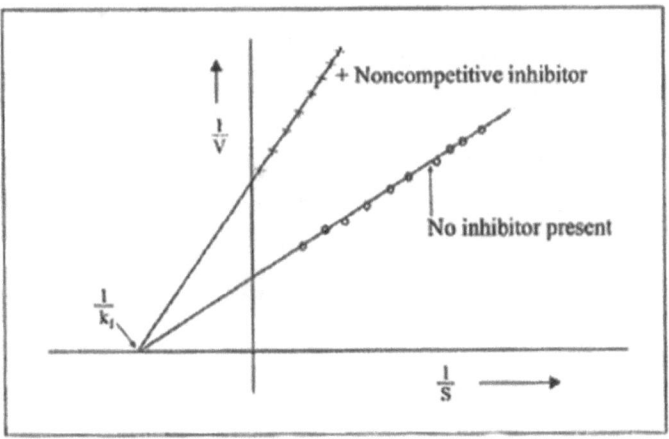

Figure 7.3: *Lineweaver-Burke plot, double-reciprocal plot of enzyme kinetic in the presence (ooo) and absence of (xxx) of non-competitor inhibitor*

A non-competitive inhibitor can combine with an enzyme molecule to produce a dead-end complex; (EI), (EIS) regardless of whether a substrate molecule is bound or not. Hence the inhibition must bind at a different site from the substrate. It is similar to the mechanism of Hyperbolic Competitive Inhibition.

We can consider special case where the inhibitor destroys the catalytic activity of the enzyme either by binding to the catalytic site or as a result of a conformational change affecting the catalytic site but does not affect the substrate binding site. The situation is as follows:

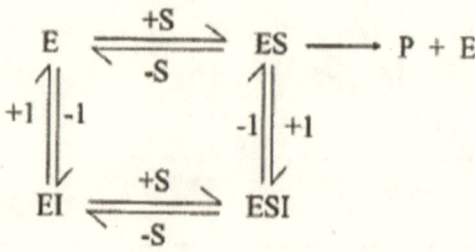

Scheme 7: *Pattern for a non-competitive inhibition*

Many types of non-competitive inhibition are consistent with the Michaelis-Menten (M–M) type equation and occur if the equilibrium assumption is valid.

In the case of the simplest linear non-competitive inhibition, the substrate does not affect inhibitor binding. Thus, under this condition, there exists the following:

Inhibitor complexes:
$$E + I \rightleftharpoons EI \quad \text{(a)}$$
$$ES + I \rightleftharpoons ESI \quad \text{(b)}$$

Inhibitor complexes:
$$E + I \rightleftharpoons EI \quad \text{(a)}$$
$$ES + I \rightleftharpoons ESI \quad \text{(b)}$$

Diagrammatically:

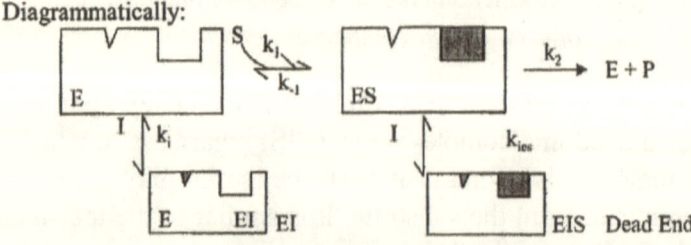

Figure 7.4: *Schematic representation of non-competitive inhibitor at the active sites of enzyme*

The dissociation constant, (Inhibitor Constant) K_i are identical in equation (a) and (b) above.

$$K_m = K_s.$$

But

$$\frac{[E][S]}{[ES]} = K_m.$$

In presence of a non-competitive inhibitor which will bind equally well to E or to ES.

$$k_1 = \frac{[E][I]}{[EI]} = \frac{[ES][I]}{[ESI]} \quad (7.9)$$

$$E_0 = [E] + [ES] + [EI] + [ESI]$$

$$E_0 = E + ES + \frac{[E)][I]}{k_i} + \frac{[ES][I]}{k_i} \quad (7.10)$$

Thus

$$E_0 = E + (ES) + \frac{(E)(I)}{k_i} + \frac{(ES)(I)}{k_i}$$

Hence,

$$(E) + (ES) = \frac{[E_0]}{1 + \frac{(I)}{k_i}} \quad (7.11)$$

$$E = \frac{[E_0]}{1 + \frac{[I]}{k_i}} - ES \quad (7.12)$$

From equation (7.7):

$$ES = \frac{E_0}{1 + \frac{K_m}{S}\left(1 + \frac{I}{k_i}\right)}$$

and

$$V_{max} = k_2 [ES].$$

Substituting for ES

$$V_0 = V_0 = \frac{V_{max}}{1 + \frac{[I_0]}{k_i}} \cdot \frac{[S_0]}{[S_0] + K_m} \qquad (7.13)$$

In non-competitive inhibition, Figure 7.5, V_{max} is reduced and so the intercept on the Y-axis is increased. The slope which is equal to K_m/V'_{max} is increased by the same factor.

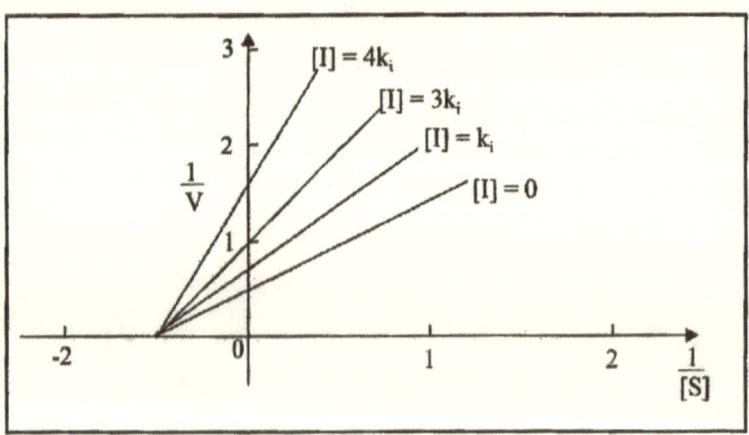

Figure 7.5: *Lineweaver-Burke plot in non-competitive inhibition*

7.3 UNCOMPETITIVE INHIBITION

The inhibitors bind only to the enzyme-substrate complex and not to the free enzyme. Substrate binding could cause a conformational change to take place in the enzyme and reveal an inhibitor binding-site.

$$(E) + (S) \underset{k_{-1}}{\overset{k_1}{\rightleftharpoons}} (ES) \overset{k_2}{\longrightarrow} E + P$$

$$\Big\updownarrow k_i$$

ESI (Dead-end complex)

$$k_i = \frac{(ES)(I)}{(ESI)} \qquad (7.14)$$

Under Steady State Condition

$$\frac{(E)(S)}{(ES)} = K_m \qquad (7.15)$$

But,

$$E_0 = (E) + (ES) + (ESI)$$

$$E_0 = (E) + (ES) + \frac{(ES)(I)}{k_i}$$

$$E_0 = (E) + (ES)\left(1 + \frac{(I)}{k_i}\right). \qquad (7.16)$$

Therefore,

$$E = (E_0) - (ES)\left(1 + \frac{(I)}{k_i}\right) \qquad (7.17)$$

But from equation (7.17)

$$ES = \frac{[E_0]}{1 + \frac{K_m}{S_0}\left(1 + \frac{I}{k_i}\right)}$$

and

$$V_{max} = k_2[ES]$$

Substituting for (E) and ES:

$$V_0 = \frac{V_{max}(S_0)}{(S_0) \times \left\{1 + \frac{(I_0)}{k_i}\right\} + K_m} \qquad (7.18)$$

Dividing numerator and denominator by $1 + \frac{(I_0)}{k_i}$

$$V_0 = \frac{\frac{V_{max}}{\left\{1 + \frac{(I_0)}{k_i}\right\}} \cdot [S_0]}{(S_0) + \frac{K_m}{\left\{1 + \frac{(I_0)}{k_i}\right\}}} \qquad (7.19)$$

If we define and

$$V'_{max} = \frac{V_{max}}{\left\{1 + \frac{(I_0)}{k_i}\right\}}$$

and

$$K'_m = \frac{K_m}{\left\{1 + \frac{(I_0)}{k_i}\right\}}$$

If V'_{max} is the apparent value of V_{max} in the presence of an initial concentration of $[I_0]$ of Uncompetitive inhibitor and K'_m is the apparent value of K_m under the same condition. The L-B equation in the presence of Uncompetitive Inhibitor is given by

$$\frac{1}{V_0} = \frac{K_m}{V'_{max}} \cdot \frac{1}{(S_0)} \times \frac{1}{V'_{max}} \qquad (7.20)$$

and the slope of the L-B plot is given as follows: (See Figure 7.6.

$$\frac{K_m}{V'_{max}} = \frac{K_m}{V_{max}} \frac{\left\{1 + \frac{(I_0)}{k_i}\right\}}{\left\{1 + \frac{(I_0)}{k_i}\right\}} \qquad (7.21)$$

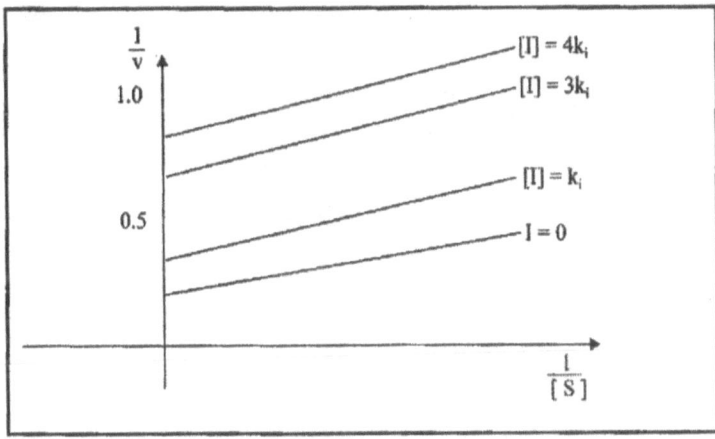

Figure 7.6 *Lineweaver-Burke plot* in Uncompetitive inhibition.

7.4 MIXED INHIBITION

In this case, the equilibrium assumption for which linear non-competitive inhibition depend does not hold, and secondly the substrate-binding and inhibitor binding are not completely independent. Generally, there are two processes by which the inhibitor may bind to the enzyme.

(i) $E + I \rightleftharpoons EI$ (Inhibitor constant,) k_i
(ii) $ES + I \rightleftharpoons ESI$ (Inhibitor constant,) k_{ies}

Thus,

$$k_i = \frac{(E)(I)}{EI}$$

and

$$k'_{ies} = -\frac{(ES)(I)}{(ESI)}.$$

And if

$$E + S \underset{k_{-1}}{\overset{K_S}{\rightleftharpoons}} ES \xrightarrow{k_2} E + P$$

$$ES + I \xrightarrow{k_{ies}} ESI$$

But for single substrate,

$$\frac{[E][S]}{[ES]} = K_m.$$

and

$$E_0 = [E] + [ES] + [EI] + [ESI].$$

If K_i is not identical with K_{ies}, k_i

$$E_0 = E + (ES) + \frac{(E)(I)}{K_i} + \frac{(ES)+(I)}{K_{ies}}$$

$$V = \frac{V_{max}[S]/(1+[I]/k_{ies})}{[S] + k_m \left(\dfrac{1+[I]/k_i}{1+[I]/k_{ies}} \right)} \quad (7.22)$$

The identical expression would be obtained if the inhibitor-binding site was separate from the substrate binding site *provided* the binding of the substrate to the enzyme resulted in the blockage of the inhibitor-binding site by a conformational change or other *mechanism*.

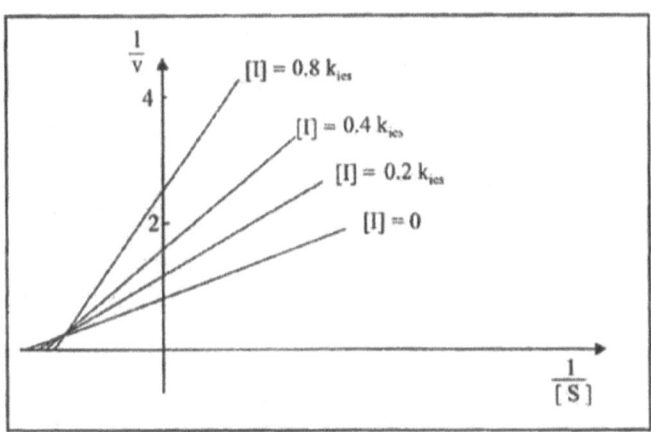

Figure 7.4: *Lineweaver-Burke plot in Non-competitive inhibition ($k_{ies} > k_i$)*

7.5 Determination of Inhibitor Constants

The inhibitor constants can be determined more accurately by graphical plots; either from the primary (double-reciprocal) or the *secondary plots*. The latter involve the plot of the *slope* or intercept values in the Primary L-B plot versus the varying inhibitor concentration in the experiment (see Figure 7.6). From the basic

Michaelis-Menten equation for the competitive inhibition; equation (7.8). The new kinetic constant, K_m' can be defined as

$$K_m' = K_m\left(1 + \frac{[I_0]}{K_i}\right)$$

$$K_m' = \frac{K_m}{K_1}.I_0 + K_m$$

where K_m', inhibitor constant, I_0, inhibitor concentration, K_m, Michaelis constant. A plot of K_m' versus $[I_0]$ is linear as shown in Figure 7.5a). Also the plot of the slope of the primary L-B plot versus $[I_0]$ is linear Figure 7.5b).

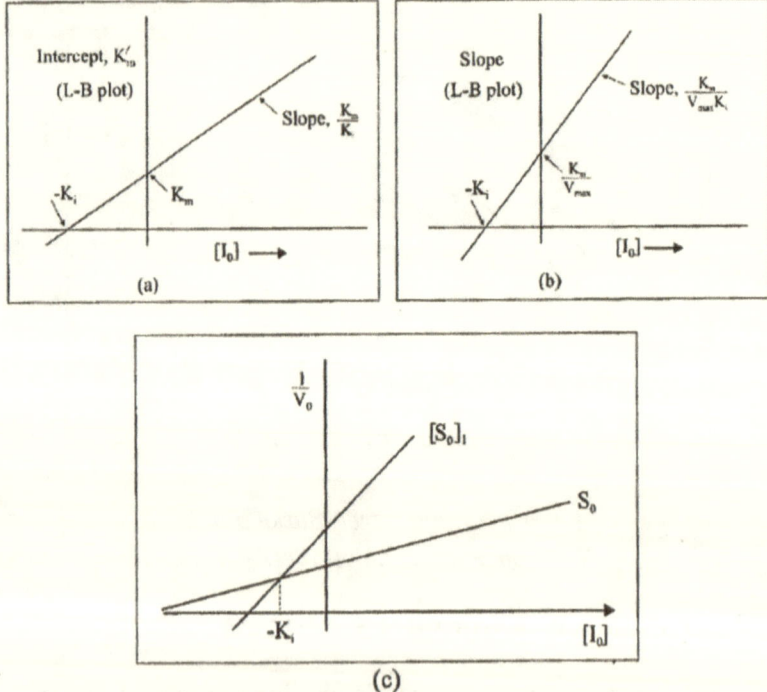

Figure 7.5:   (a) *Plot of intercept against inhibitor concentration*
              (b) *Plot of slope against inhibitor concentration*
              (c) *Dixon Plot.*

ESSENTIALS OF ENZYMOLOGY

Dixon has suggested another plot for obtaining the Inhibitor constant. This is derived from the Basic Equation, (equation 7.8). On inverting the equation (7.8) we find

$$\frac{1}{V_0} = \frac{K_m \left(1 + \frac{[I_0]}{k_i} \times \frac{1}{[S_0]}\right)}{V_{max}} + \frac{1}{V_{max}}$$

Hence,

$$\frac{1}{V_0} = \frac{K_m \times [I_0]}{V_{max}[S_0]k_i} + \frac{K_m}{V_{max}[S_0]} + \frac{1}{V_{max}}$$

At fixed substrate concentration [S] the plot of $\frac{1}{V_0}$ versus $[I_0]$ gives straight lines which intersect at the 3rd quadrangle, see Figure 7.5(c). This is referred to as the *Dixon plot*. From this plot, the inhibitor constant can be obtained.

In the above cases, the primary and secondary plots are linear, hence this situation is referred to as *Linear Competitive Inhibition*. For complicated systems, the primary plots may be linear while the secondary plots are non-linear. The other conditions which are often seen in inhibition assays include:

(i) *Parabolic Competitive Inhibition* in which the shape of the Dixon plot and the secondary plots are parabolas.
(ii) *Hyperbolic Competitive Inhibition* in which the inhibitor binds to a different site from the substrate and reduces the affinity of the enzyme for the substrate without altering the reaction characteristics of that substrate which also binds to the enzyme.

7.6 SUMMARY

Four patterns of enzyme inhibition can be recognised namely:

(i)   Competitive Inhibition
(ii) Uncompetitive Inhibition
(iii) Classic Noncompetitive Inhibition
(iv) Mixed-Non Competitive Inhibition-(Mixed Inhibitor)

The characteristics of the different types of the reverse enzyme inhibition are provided in Table 7.1.

Table 7.1: *Characteristics of different types of reversible enzyme inhibition*

Type of Inhibition	Inhibitor combines with	Effect on V_{max}	Effect on K_m	Effect on $\dfrac{1}{V_0}$ against $\dfrac{1}{[S]}$ plot
1. Competitive	E	Unchanged	Increased	Convergence on ordinate axis
2. Uncompetitive	ES	Decreased	Decreased	Parallel lines
3. Non-competitive (i) Simple, $K_i = K_{ies}$	"E" and "ES"	Decreased	Unchanged	Convergence on abscissa
(ii) Mixed, $K_{ies} > K_i$		Decreased	Increased	Convergence above abscissa
(iii) Mixed, $K_{ies} < K_i$		Decreased	Increased	Convergence below abscissa

The graphical pattern of the kinetics for each type of Inhibition are illustrated by the Lineweaver - Burke (L-B) plot and Eadie-Hofstee plots.

ESSENTIALS OF ENZYMOLOGY

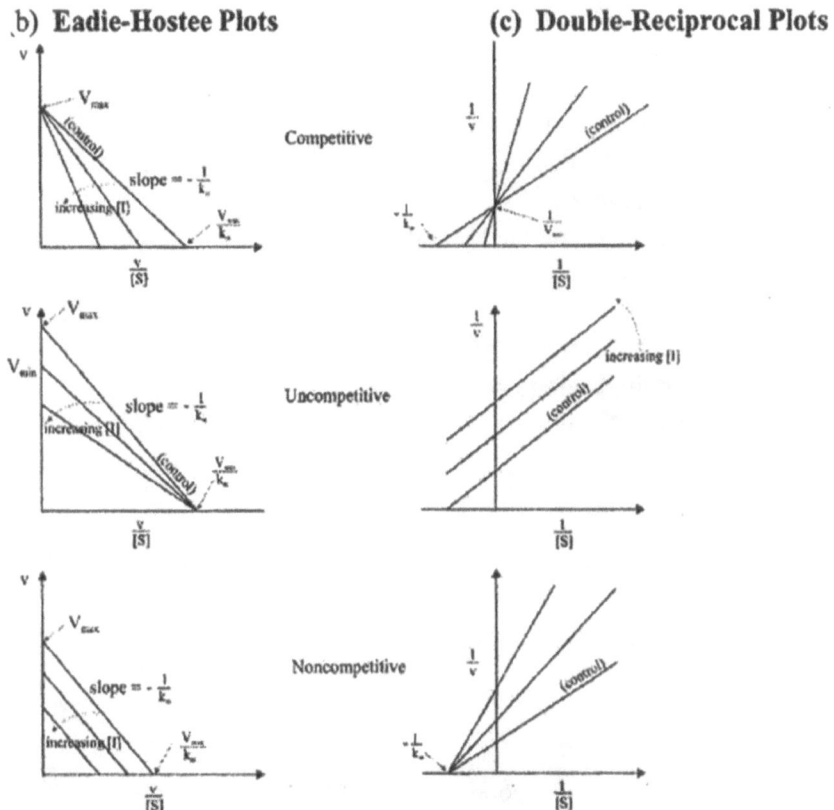

Figure 7.6: *Patterns of Enzyme Inhibition Kinetics (Double reciprocal and Eadie-Hostee), I = inhibitor, S = substrate and v = initial velocity*

REVIEW QUESTIONS *(Enzymes Kinetics)*

1. Describe the relationship between the kinetic constants and the equilibrium constant of a reversible enzyme reaction.
2. What do you understand by the term "Steady State" as applied in enzyme kinetics? Derive the Briggs-Haldane equation for the "steady state" condition.
3. Write notes on:
   Fast Reaction Techniques
   Ping-Pong Mechanism in enzyme kinetics
   Non-Competitive Inhibition
   Cooperativity Effects.

4. Discuss briefly the diagnostic parameters, which can be employed to distinguish the major mechanisms in multi-substrate reactions.
5. Outline 4 different possibilities for mechanisms of two-substrate enzyme catalyzed reactions in terms of how the individual steps may be formulated.
6. Enumerate the major types of enzyme inhibition patterns and give examples.
7. What type of enzyme mechanism gives non-linear primary plots of 1/v versus 1/s? Give reasons for this phenomenon.
8. Malate dehydrogenase catalyzes the reaction:
   L-malate + NAD^+ ------------> Oxaloacetate + NADH + H^+

The rate of the forward reaction was investigated in the presence of saturations of malate and a fixed concentration of enzyme. The following results were obtained:

NAD^+ concn. Absorbance (at 340 nm) at time t (mins)

Mmol.l^{-1}	t=0.5	1.0	1.5	2.0	2.5	3.0
1.5	0.33	0.056	0.079	0.102	0.122	0.138
2.0	0.036	0.063	0.089	0.116	0.138	0.154
2.5	0.040	0.069	0.099	0.128	0.150	0.168
3.33	0.043	0.075	0.108	0.140	0.163	0.175
5.0	0.047	0.084	0.121	0.158	0.177	0.184
10.0	0.052	0.095	0.137	-.180	0.192	0.20

Calculate Km and Vmax.

9. Five reaction mixtures containing equal concentrations of an enzyme are made up to the substrate concentrations indicated in the Table 1.1 below; and the initial rates of reaction are measured. The experiment is then repeated with an enzyme inhibitor at a concentration of $2.2 \times 10^{-4}M$ in each reaction mixture:

(i) Using Line weaver-Burk plots of these data, graphically determine K_m for the substrate, K_i for the inhibitor, and Vmax in the absence and presence of inhibitor

(ii) Is this a competitive or non-competitive inhibitor?

Table 1.I: *Initial Rates at various substrate concentrations in the presence and absence of an inhibitor for an enzyme-catalysed reaction*

(S) (Moles/Litre)	Inhibitor absent V: (Umoles/Min)	Inhibitor Present - 2.2×10^{-4}M V: (Umoles/Min)
1.0×10^{-4}	28	18
1.5×10^{-4}	36	24
2.0×10^{-4}	43	30
5.0×10^{-4}	63	51
7.5×10^{-4}	74	63

10. The activity of a glycosidase is inhibited by an acid. The initial velocity of the hydrolysis of the glycoside, as determined by the release of reducing sugar, is measured under varying conditions of glycoside and inhibitor concentration. The level of glycosidase is constant. The results are given in Table 2.

Determine the type of inhibition and the values of K_{ii}, K_{is}, K_m, and the maximum velocity, V_{max}.

Table 2

Inhibitor	Glycoside (Cleaved in Umole/2min)		
(I) (nM) at	(S) = 6.25mM at	(S) – 0, 862mM	(S) – 0.42mM
0.0	0.625	0.455	0.340
1.0	0.488	0.352	0.265
2.0	0.400	0.289	0.217
3.0	0.399	0.244	0.184
4.0	0.294	0.213	0.159

REFERENCES

A. ENZYME KINETICS I & II

1. Briggs, G.E. and Haldane, J.B.S. (1925). *Biochem. J.* 19, 338.
2. Eadie G.S. (1942). *J. Biol. Chem.* 146. 85
3. Dalziel, K. (1969). *Biochem. J.* 114, 547-556.
4. Cleland, W.W. (1963). *Biochim. Biophys. Acta* 67. 188-196.
5. Wong, J.T.F. and Hanes C.S (1962). *Can J. Biochem. & Physiology* 40, 763.
6. Cleland, W.W. (1967). *Adv. Enzymol.* 29, 1-32
7. Michaelis, L and Menten, M.L. (1913). *Biochem. Zeitschr.* 49, 333-369.
8. Hill, A.V. (1913). *Biochem. J.* 7, 471-480.
9. Koshland, D.E. & Nemethyl G. and Filmer (1966). *Biochem.* 5. 365-385
10. Monod, J., Wyman J., & Changeux J.P. (1965). *J. Mol. Biol.* 12, 88-118.

B. ENZYME INHIBITION

1. Williams, J.W. Duggleby, R.G. Cutler, R and Morrison, J. F. (1980). *Biochem Pharmacol.* 29. 589-591
2. Schloss, J.V. Porter, D.J.T. Bright, H.J and Cleland, W.W. (1980). *Biochemistry.* 19. 2358-2362
3. Viola, R.E. Morrison, J.F & Cleland W.W. (1980). *Biochemistry* 19, 3131-3137
4. Rich, D.H. and Sun, E.T.O. (1980). *Biochemistry Pharmacol.* 29, 2205-2212.
5. Neet, K.E. and Ainslie, G.R. (1980). *Meth. Enzymol.* 64. 192-226.

C. SUGGESTIONS FOR FURTHER READING

1. Engel, P.C. (ed.) (1981). *Enzyme Kinetics. The Steady-State Approach.* 2nd edn. CHAPMAN & HALL
2. Ainsworth, Stanley (ed) *Steady-State Enzyme Kinetics:* (Macmillian)

3. Davies, E.A. (1980). *Quantitative Biochemistry.* 6th edn. Longman, (Chps 3-6)
4. Trevor Palmer (ed) (1976). *Understanding Enzymes-(Horwood* Publishing Coy. Chemistry.
5. Trevor Palmer (ed) (2001). *Enzymes- Biochemistry, Biotechnology, Clinical Chemistry.* (Norwood Publishing Coy.)
6. Cornish-Bowden A (ed) (1995). *Fundamentals of Enzyme kinetics* 2nd edn. Portland Press. (Chapter 5)
7. Choudhary, M.I ed. (1996). *Biological Inhibitors.* Harwood Academic Publishers.
8. Price, N.C. and Stevens, L. (1999). *Fundamentals of Enzymology,* 3rd edn. Oxford University Press, (Chapter 4).
9. Gutfreund, H. (1999). "Rapid flow techniques and their Contributions to enzymology". *Trends in Biochemical Science* 24, 457-460.
10. Segel, I.H. (1975). reissued (1993) *Enzyme Kinetics,* Wiley, (Chapter 6,9,10.)
11. Dixton, M. Webb E.C. et al. (1979). *Enzymes* 3rd edn. Longman, Chapter 4.

PART III
Enzyme Catalysis, Mechanism And Regulation

CHAPTER EIGHT

Enzyme Catalysis And Mechanisms

8.0 INTRODUCTION

Catalysis involves the breaking and formation of bonds Thus, the understanding of a chemical reaction, (enzymes or not) entails the knowledge of the bonds broken and formed and the nature of the intermediates, if any produced in the course of the reaction.

There are four common features of enzyme catalysis that can be recognised:

(i) The rates, that is, (turnover number), of enzyme reactions do not vary greatly despite the very great variety in the types of chemical reactions. The rates of enzyme-catalysed reactions can be divided into two classes (a) reactions involving only electron transfer. (b) reactions involving both electron and proton (hydrogen) transfer. Under optimal conditions; the turnover number of reactions of class (b) is approximately 10^3 moles of substrate/mol. of enzyme; whereas that of class (a) is roughly 10^8.

(ii) Chemical catalysis by enzyme proteins is mediated by a limited number of different functional groups. The inert side chains of the amino acids: alanine, phenylalanine, leucine, valine, proline, isoleucine are not involved in the catalysis. Of the remaining, a number are of similar types, thus,: glutamic acid/aspartic acid; threonine/serine and asparagine/glutamine. Hence, the chemical "elements" for the construction of a catalytic site

are highly restricted. The side-chain residues of histidine are involved in the catalytic process of a variety of enzymes.
(iii) The rates of enzyme-catalysed reactions show a pH-dependent optimum which is fairly close to pH 7.
(iv) Many enzyme molecules are very large in comparison to their substrates.

The major types of catalytic chemical processes which are also found in enzyme catalysed reactions include acid/base catalysis, nucleophilic/electrophilic catalysis (covalent catalysis) and metal-ion catalysis.

8.1 ACID-BASE CATALYSIS

The catalysis of reaction by acids and bases is a general phenomenon in organic chemistry. Acid-base catalysis can be divided into two major categories based on empirical observations:

(i) specific acid and specific base catalysis;
(ii) general acid and general base catalysis.

The specific base or acid catalysis involves reactions whose rates vary in a linear fashion with hydroxyl (OH^-) or hydrogen (H^+ ion concentrations), but do not vary with the concentration of other acidic or basic species. On the other hand, the general acid or general base catalysis is associated with reactions whose rates are a function of the concentration of all species. If the concept of acids is extended to include non-protonic compounds- that are capable of co-ordinating with an unshared electron pair (Lewis acids); the concept of general acid catalysis may also be extended to include catalysis by such acids particularly *metal-ion* (superacid catalysis). The efficiency of a particular species as a general acid or general base catalysis is primarily a function of its acid or base strength. This statement is expressed quantitatively in the Bronsted Catalysis Law.

$$\kappa_A = G_A (K)^\alpha \qquad (1)$$

$$\kappa_B = G_B\left(\frac{1}{K}\right)^\beta \qquad (2)$$

Whereby, κ_A and κ_B are the catalytic constants for acid and base catalysis respectively;

K is the dissociation constant of the acid catalyst or the conjugate acid of the base catalyst;. G_B, G_A, α, β are constants that depend on the nature of the reaction, the solvent and the temperature.

The magnitude of the exponents, a and b in the Bronsted catalysis laws measures indirectly the susceptibility of the reaction to general acid-base catalysis.

Therefore,

$$\log \kappa_A = \log G_A - \alpha pK_a, \qquad (3)$$

$$\log \kappa_B = \log G_B - \beta pK_b. \qquad (4)$$

Hence

1. The plots of catalytic constants against corresponding values of pKa yield straight lines whose slopes define the magnitude of α and β.
2. These exponents are by definition, positive and take values between 0 and unity (1).
3. The magnitude of the exponent measures the sensitivity of a reaction rate to changes in the strength of the catalyzing acid or base. Large values indicates a high sensitivity and small values indicating a relative insensitivity.

    (i) If α value is 1; the reaction is highly sensitive to the strength of the acid catalyst and H^+ is the only effective catalyst detectable.
    (ii) If α value is near zero, it indicates all acids are of approximate equal efficiency, as catalysis.

Biochemical reactions which are susceptible to acid-base catalysis include (a) carbonyl addition reactions (b) hydrolysis of some carboxylic or phosphoric esters (c) aminolysis of esters (d) tautomerizations.

The typical reactions of the above are enumerated below:

Table: 8.0 *Some Examples of Reactions Exhibiting Acid-Base Catalysis*

	Reaction	Type of catalysis
(i)	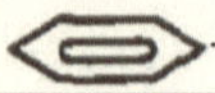 Ph–CHO + $NH_2 \cdot NH \cdot COO \cdot NH_2$	General acid
(ii)	Glucose Mutarotation	General acid/general base
(iii)	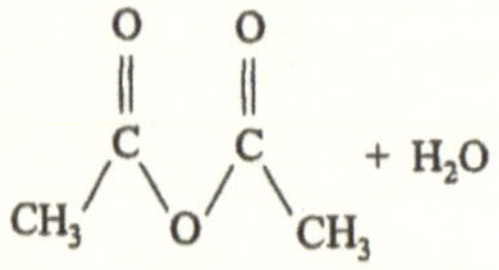 $CH_3-CO-O-CO-CH_3 + H_2O$	General base
(iv)	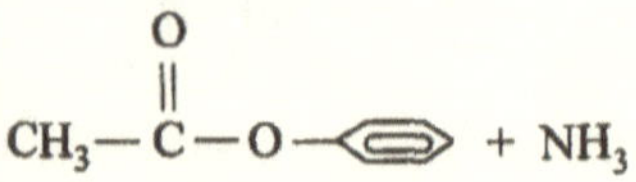 $CH_3-C(=O)-O-Ph + NH_3$	General base
(v)	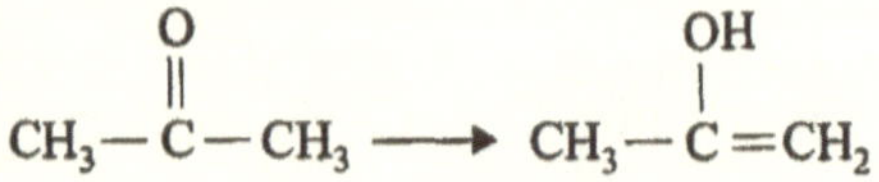 $CH_3-C(=O)-CH_3 \longrightarrow CH_3-C(OH)=CH_2$	General acid, general base.

8.2 NUCLEOPHILIC AND ELECTROPHILIC CATALYSIS [COVALENT CATALYSIS]

Nucleophiles are molecules or anions in which one atom has an unshared pair of electrons which it can readily share with an electron - deficient atom in another molecule to form a covalent bond. The latter molecule is defined as an *electrophile,* it has an atom capable of accepting a share in a pair of electron. The general scheme illustrating the basic concept is shown below.

Hence;

$$E + :N \longrightarrow E-N \xrightarrow{\text{nucleophilic catalysis}} \text{product} + :N \qquad [1]$$

$$\xrightarrow{\text{electrophilic catalysis}} \text{product} + E \qquad [2]$$

Thus, an atomic centre which has a strong tendency to donate an electron pair is termed a *nucleophile*. Likewise, a catalysed reaction that proceeds via the donation of an electron-pair from the catalyst to the substrate is termed *nucleophilic catalysis*.

The essential feature of a nucleophile or electrophile catalyst is that it reacts with the substrate to form an intermediate which then reacts further to give the final products and regenerate the catalyst. Thus, this mode of catalysis is generally referred to as *covalent catalysis*. It is characterised by the existence of a covalently-bond substrate-catalyst intermediate.

Examples of nucleophiles include, -OH (serine), -SH (cysteine), $-CO_2$ (aspartate), $-NH_2$ (lysine), imidazole (histidine) and aromatic hydroxyl group (tyrosine). Increasingly large numbers of enzyme-catalysed reactions are known to occur with covalent catalysis. The typical reactions include (a) decarboxylation of the acetoacetic acid, (b) pyridoxal phosphate and (c) thiamine pyrophosphate catalysed reactions. These involve substrates at the acyl level of oxidation that are subject to nucleophilic catalysis. Also, the imidazole - catalysed acyl transfer and hydrolysis reaction which occur via the intermediate formation of acyl imidazoles. Generally, enzymatic reactions which occur via a nucleophile route, hence are subject to nucleophilic catalysis include:

(i) substrates at the aldehyde level of oxidation;
(ii) semi-carbazone formation from pyridoxal and pyridoxal phosphate with both primary and secondary amines;
(iii) carbonyl addition reactions;
(iv) activation of the carbon atom β to the carbonyl group;
(v) reactions involving substrates at the acyl level of oxidation.

The factors that influence nucleophilicites include the following::

(a) basicity of the attacking reagent(s);
(b) abnormally high polarizabilities ion, such as peroxide anion, and sulfhydryl anion;
(c) steric effects;
(d) solvation effects;
(e) compounds with an unshared electron pair adjacent to the attacking atom. In this case, nucleophilic catalysis has been attributed to the donation of electron to the attacking in the transition state.

8.3 METAL-ION CATALYSIS

Over 25% of all enzymes contain tightly bound metal ions or require them for activity. The functions of these metals studied by X-ray crystallography and electron spin resonance (ESR), have provided insight into the roles of metals ions in enzymatic catalysis. There are two major classes: namely (a) metalloenzymes which contain a definite quantity of functional metal ion that is retained throughout purification, (b) metal activated enzymes which bind metals less tightly but require added metals. The mechanisms of action in both groups are very similar.

Generally, metal ions facilitate substrate binding and catalysis. Metals function in catalysis by the formation of a ternary (3 components) complex of the catalytic site (ENZ), a metal ion [M] and substrate [S] that exhibit 1:1:1. stoichiometry. Thus, four (4) schemes are possible:

(a) Enz - S - M - [Substrate-bridge-complex]
(b) M -= Enz – S- [Enzymes-bridge complex]
(c) Enz - M - S - [Simple-metal-bridge complex]
(d) $Enz \bigg\langle \genfrac{}{}{0pt}{}{M}{\underset{S}{|}}$: cyclic - metal bridge complex

Whilst, all the four kinds are possible with metal activated enzymes; the metalloenzymes cannot form the substrate bridge complex. Metal ions, like protons are Lewis acids (electrophiles) that can store an electron pair, forming a sigma bond. They can also accept electrons via sigma or pi bonds to activate electrophiles or nucleophiles (general acids/base catalysis). By donating electrons, metal can activate nucleophiles or act as nucleophiles themselves. The coordination sphere of a metal brings together enzyme and substrate (approximation) to form chelate; producing distortion in either the enzymes or substrate (strain). Also, metals can serve as 3- dimensional templates for orientation of basic groups on the enzyme or substrate.

8.4 ENZYME MECHANISMS

General Consideration

The mechanisms for most of the enzymes whose crystal structures have been solved at high resolution of X-ray crystallography are now well-documented. These include the dehydrogenases (alcohol dehydrogenase, lactate dehydrogenase, glyceraldehyde-3-phosphate dehydrogenase); proteases, (serine proteases; thiol-proteases; carboxypeptidases); ribonuclease, staphylococcal nuclease, lysozyme; carbonic anhydrase; glycolytic enzymes (triose phosphate isomerase, glucose - 6- phosphate isomerase, phosphoglycerate mutase.

The contributions to the enzyme catalysis as formulated from the chemical studies on any enzyme can be attributed to the following factors, general acid-base catalysis; metal-ion catalysis, nucleophilic catalysis, electrostatic catalysis, propinquity effects (a combination of an intramolecular reaction and correct orientation, strain distortion of substrate; induced - fit (distortion of enzyme).

The general acid-base catalysis is the most ubiquitous being found in the reactions of the dehydrogenases, the serine proteinases and most probably the thiol proteases and carboxypeptidase, ribonuclease, lysozyme and the aldose-ketose isomerases. The metal-ion catalysis which involves stabilisation of an anion, is found in the mechanisms of carboxypeptidase and possibly alcohol dehydrogenase. Nucleophilic catalysis occurs during the hydrolysis catalysed by the thiol and serine proteases and also in the reactions of many enzymes where schiff bases are formed between the carbonyl group of the substrate and the side chain of a lysine residue.

Electrostatic catalysis is important in the stabilization of the carbonium ion intermediate in the reactions of lysozyme. There is no direct evidence for the distortion of substrate on being bound to an enzyme and propinquity effects are not easily studied. However, examples of strain in the form of "transition-state stabilization" and also distortion of the enzyme on binding a substrate have been reported.

A short description on mechanism of catalysis on two specific enzymes that may provide an exciting insight into the chemical basis of enzyme catalysis will be discussed below.

8.5 CHYMOTRYPSIN

This is a small extracellular enzyme with molecular mass of about 25,000. It contains 245 amino acids in a single polypeptide chain. It is an endopeptidase which belongs to the group, serine proteases, that have a reactive serine residue and pH optima around neutrality. The serine proteases catalyse the hydrolysis of ester or amide substrates.

The α-chymotrypsin molecule is roughly spherical and extremely compact, with the main polypeptide chain folded closely back upon one another. Folding is rather irregular, although there are some short lengths of β-sheet secondary structure, and a small of α-helix, of which, the sequence from residues 234 - 245 is the most visible. The enzyme requires no metal ions or co-factors for its activity.

The hydrolysis of esters or amide substrates involves an acyl enzyme intermediate in which the hydroxyl group of *Ser - 195* is acylated by the substrate. The formation of the acyl-enzyme is the slow step in the reaction of saturating concentrations of amide substrates but the acyl-enzyme often accumulates in the hydrolysis of esters.

(a) Substrate-Binding Site of Chymotrypsin

In the three-dimensional structure of the enzyme, the substrate binding site is close to the uniquely reactive *Serine - 195*. The site is a deep but has narrow pocket created by the folding of the enzyme chain lined with largely hydrophobic residues. This is designed to accommodate the non-polar side-chains of a typical substrate; and this favours interaction needed as the driving force. For the substrate-binding specifically, studies indicate that a second favourable interaction involves the acyl-amino portion of the substrate, and from the crystal structure, this can be identified as a hydrogen bond to the carbonyl group of the Serine - 124. The susceptible carbonyl group points towards the main-chain peptide groups of both Gly - 193 and Ser - 195 which play an important role in the catalytic process.

(b) The Charge-Relay System for Chymotrypsin

The active site of chymotrypsin can be located in the three dimensional structure as a shallow depression on the enzyme surface next to the substrate binding site. As the chemical studies predicted, it contains both Serine - 195 and Histidine -57: The hydroxyl group of the serine is sufficiently close to the imidazole ring of the histidine that it forms a hydrogen bond to one of the ring nitrogen atoms. The second ring nitrogen is in turn hydrogen-bonded to the negatively-charged carboxylate group of Aspartic acid - 102 which lies directly behind it, completely screened from the solvent and in a rather hydrophobic environment.

The Aspartic acid - 102 acts as a general base, thus protonation of the buried negative charges takes place. This catalytic process so called charge-relay system, is outlined in Figure 8.1.

The nucleophilic attack by Ser - 195 on a peptide substrate leads first to an unstable adduct with a tetrahedral geometry. As the tetrahedral intermediate collapses to the acyl-enzyme; proton transfer from the charge-relay system allows the amine to depart as a neutral species, and restores His - 57 and Asp - 102 to their original ionisation state, see Figure 8.1.

In the next step, a water molecule will attack the carbonyl group and bring about de-acylation Figure 8.1. The rate of initial attack by *Serine - 195* determines the overall rate of hydrolysis for peptide substrates. This step is assisted in at least three ways; by the use of precise binding interactions to orient the reaction components in the optimal position for reaction; by the operation of the charge-relay system (proton-relay system) and by the stabilisation of the transition state in which negative charge develops on the carbonyl oxygen atom, through perfectly placed hydrogen bonds from the main-chain peptide nitrogen atoms of *Glycine - 193* and *Serine - 195*.

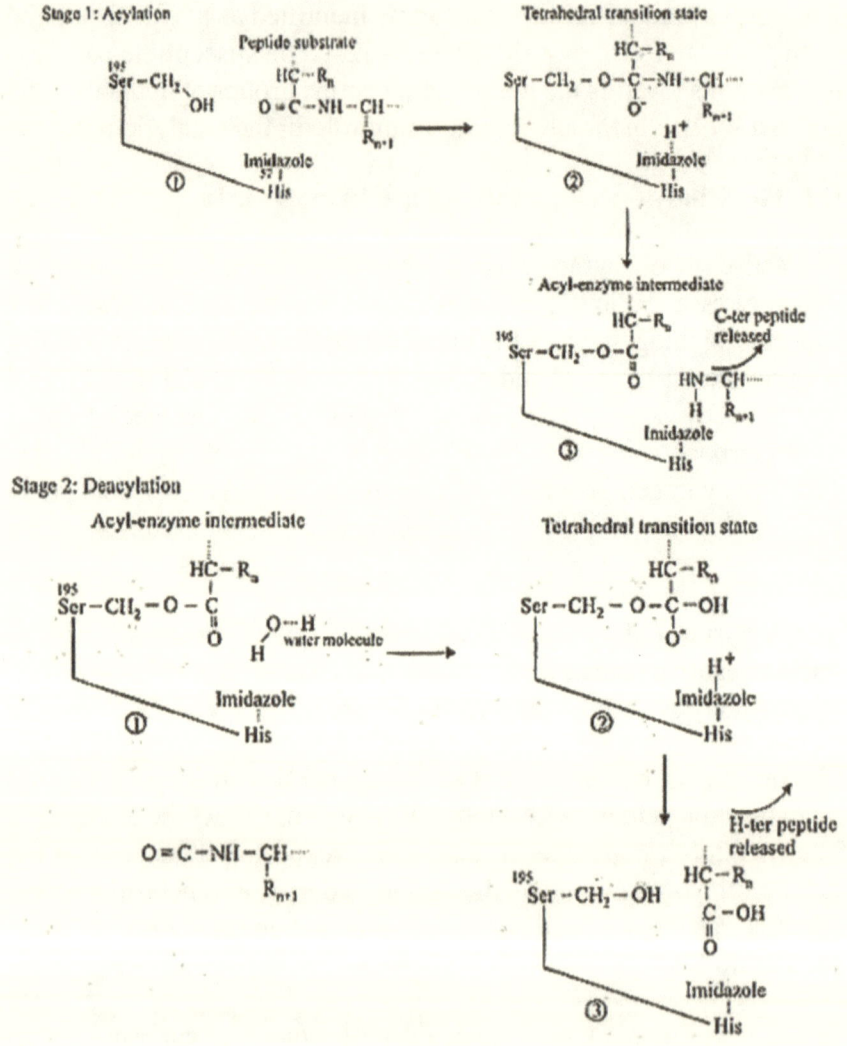

Figure 8.1: *Catalytic mechanism of serine proteinases (chymotrypsin)*

8.6 LYSOZYME

Hen egg-white lysozyme is a small protein of molecular weight 14,500 and contains 129 amino acid residues. The enzyme dissolves certain bacteria by cleaving the polysaccharide component of their cell walls. The cell wall polysaccharide is made of two kinds of sugars: N-acetylglucosamine (NAG) and N-acetylneuraminic acid (NAM). The NAM and NAG alternate in sequence. All the glycosidic bonds of the cell-wall polysaccharide have a β-configuration; hence, the cell-wall polysaccharide is an alternating polymer of NAM and NAG residues joined by β (1 → 4) glycosidic linkages. Different polysaccharide chains are cross-linked by short peptides that are attached to some of the NAM residues.

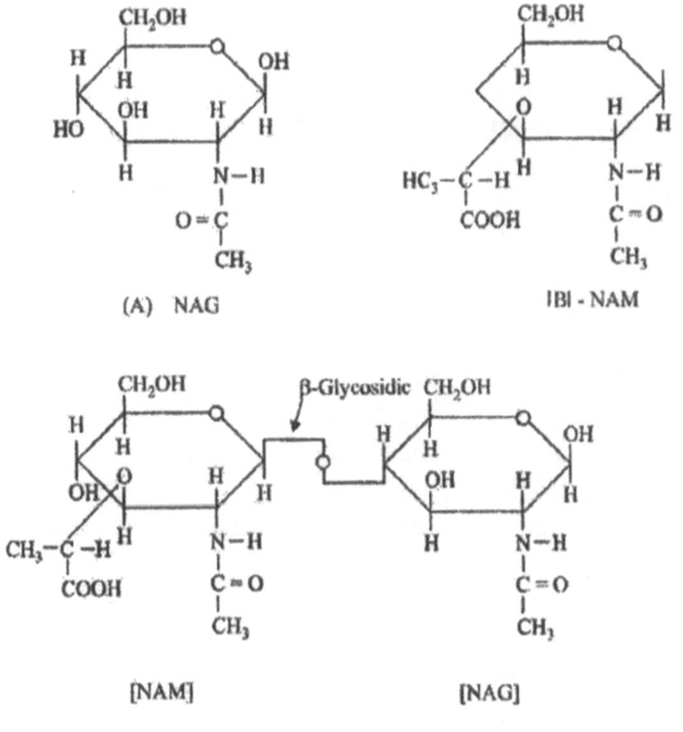

Figure 8.2: *Structures of N-acetylglucosamine (A) and N– acetylneuraminic Acid (B)*

Lysozyme hydrolyses the glycosidic bond between C - 1 of NAM and C - 4 of NAG. The other glycosidic bond between C - 1 of NAG and C - 4 of NAM is not cleaved. Chitin, polysaccharide found in the shell of crustaceans is also a substrate for lysozyme. Chitin consists only of NAG residues joined by β (1 → 4) glycosidic links. A mechanism was proposed for the enzymic reaction based on the structure of the active site and findings from physico-chemical studies of model compounds.

This consists of the following points: There are six subsites for binding the glucopyranose rings of the synthetic substrate, labelled, ABCDEF. The scissile bond lies between sites D and E close to the carboxyl groups of Glu- 35 and Asp-52. It is suggested that the reaction proceeds via a carbonium ion intermediate which is stabilised by the ionized carboxylate of Asp-52; the expulsion of the alcohol is general acid catalyzed by the unionized carboxyl of Glu-35.

Philips and his colleagues have proposed a detailed catalytic mechanism for lysozyme.

The essential steps of this proposed catalytic mechanism for Lysozyme are as follows:

(i) The -COOH group of Glutamic acid - 35 donates an H^+ to the bond between C - 1 of the bond between C - 1 of the D ring and the glycosidic oxygen atom thereby cleaving this bond (Figure 8.3).
(ii) This creates a positive charge on C - 1 of the D-ring. This transient species is called a "carbonium" ion because it contains a positively charged carbon atom.
(iii) The dimer of NAG consisting of residues E - F diffuses away from the enzyme.
(iv) The carbonium-ion intermediate then reacts with OH^- from the solvent. Tetra - NAG consisting of residues A-B-C-D diffuses away from the enzyme.
(v) Glutamic-35 becomes protonated and the enzyme is ready for another round of catalysis.

Essentially, a combination of substrate strain and acid-base catalysis is effected in the mechanism of lysozyme action, (Figure 8.4), Ring D of the hexasaccharide substrate upon binding to the enzyme is strained to the half-chair conformation. General acid catalysis by active site glutamic acid promotes the unstable half-chair into the transition state. The carbonium ion formed in the transition state is stabilised by a negatively charged aspartate. Breakage of the glycosidic linkage between rings D and E relieves the strained transition state by allowing rings D and E to return to the stable chair conformation.

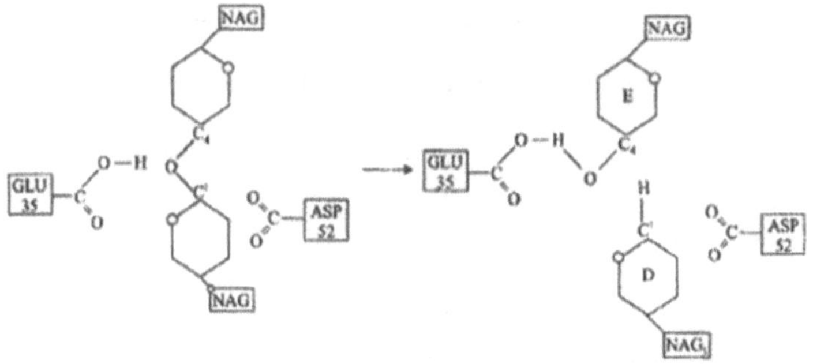

Figure 8.3: *First step in the proposed catalytic mechanism for lysozyme*

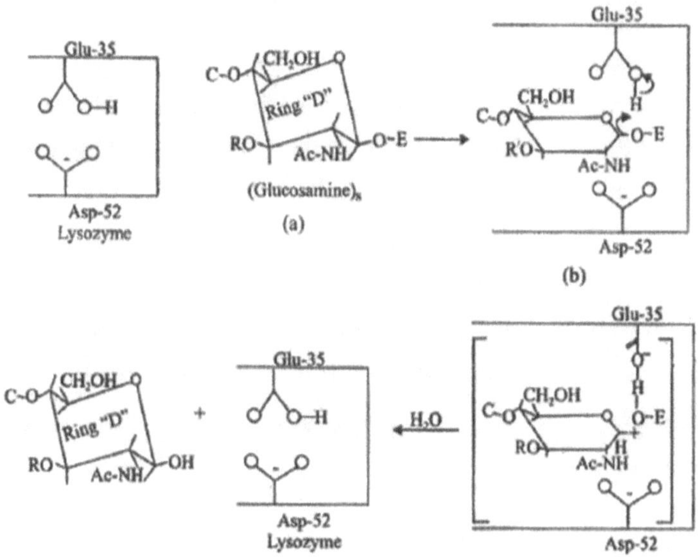

Figure 8.4: *A mechanism for lysozyme action*

The binding of the stable chair (a) conformation of the substrate to the enzyme generates the strained half-chair conformation (b) in the ES complex.

CHAPTER NINE

Active Site Of Enzymes

9.0 GENERAL CONSIDERATION

Most enzymatic reactions involve substrates that are small compared to the size of the catalyst molecule. Consequently, only a small portion of the amino acid side chains and peptide bonds are near or in direct contact with the substrate molecule in the enzyme - substrate complex. This realisation gives rise to the concept of an *active site* for enzymatic reactions. The *active site* of an enzyme is taken to include those side chains and peptide bonds which are in direct physical contact with the substrate (perhaps through intervening water molecules) and other side chains or peptide bonds that, although not in direct contact with the substrate, perform a direct function in the catalytic process. Part or all of the remainder of the protein molecule serves the less direct function of providing a structural backbone suitable for maintaining the components of the active site in the three dimensional conformation so required for efficient specific catalysis.

9.1 IDENTIFICATION OF AMINO ACIDS AT THE ACTIVE SITE OF ENZYMES

The identification of amino acids present at the active site of enzymes is clearly of major importance for the understanding of the basic facets of the mechanism of enzyme-catalysed reactions. Several methods of varying utility have been employed in attempts to identify at least some of the residues that constitute the active site. The protein group-specific reagents for identification of these residues are stated in Table 9.1.

The most direct method is to attach a covalent label which itself is stable to procedures required to degrade polypeptide chains, to some residue present in the active site. On this basis, two classes of enzymes can be distinguished; those which involve covalent enzyme-substrate intermediates in the course of catalytic process and those which do not. These labels are also called *site-specific reagents*. Three categories of these labels (reagents) can be recognised. These are (a) substrate labels, (b) pseudo-substrate labels and (c) affinity labels.

Table 9.1: *Protein Group Specific Reagents*

Protein Group	Reagent
Amino (lysine and amino terminal)	Ethyl thiotrifluoracetate
	Maleic anhydride
	Citaconic anhydride
	Methyl acetimidate/HCl
	Salicylaldehyde
	2-Methoxy-5-nitrotropone
Phenolic (tyrosine)	Succinic anhydride, Tetranitromethane
	Acetic anhydride, Iodine,
	Dinitrofluoro benzene (DNFB)
Imidazole (histidine)	Ethoxyformic anhydride; diazonium-l-H tetrazole,
Thioether (methionine)	Cyanogen bromide
	Hydrogen peroxide, a-haloketones
Sulfhydryl (Cysteine)	Mercurials;
	Disulfides;5,5'-dithiobis (2-nitro-benzoic acid));DTNB
	N- Ethylmaleimide; Sulfite
	Dinitrofluorobenzene, [DNFB}
Disulfide bridges (cystine)	Thiols; Performic acid.
	Borohydride
Guanidino (arginine)	Phenylglyoxal; Nitromalondialdehyde

9.2 SUBSTRATE LABELS

The enzyme's substrate is a perfect example of a site-specific protein reagent. The bonds between enzyme and their substrates are usually labile and transitory; however the specificity of their combination has prompted some attempts to stabilise these linkages.

For example, Acetoacetate decarboxylase enzyme when incubated with its substrate, acetoacetate and the reaction is treated with sodium borohydride, leads to the identification of lysine residue within the active site of the enzyme. This has been demonstrated by the specific labelling of one lysyl residue in the enzyme protein with the loss of catalytic activity. Similar results have been obtained with other enzymes and their specific substrates. A single lysine residue is labelled by sodium borohydride reduction of the aldolase - dihydroxyacetone phosphate complex intermediate. The labelled residues have been isolated as peptides after enzyme/chemical cleavage of the protein, and the amino acids adjacent to the labelled residues have been determined. The amount of substrate introduced in such an experiment can be used as an estimate of the number of active sites.

9.3 PSEUDO-SUBSTRATE LABELS

The reagents are so called pseudo-substrate labels on the basis of certain characteristics they are presumed to share with substrates of the enzymes under reference. For example, the serine proteases and certain esterases are inactivated by diisopropyl fluorophosphate (DIPF) through its reaction with specific serine hydroxyl group in each case. Similar amino acid sequences have been found around the reactive seryl residues in most of these enzymes. Serine itself, and serine residues in other proteins do not react under the same conditions. The special reactivity is a function of the native structure of the serine protease enzyme and is abolished upon denaturation. Certain organophosphates react similarly, with characteristically different rates with different enzymes.

Table 9.2: *Examples of some affinity labels*

Enzyme	(Reagent LABEL)	Residue modified
Aspartate aminotransferase	β-Bromopyruvate	Cystine
	β-Chloroalanine	Lysine
Carboxypeptidase B	α-N-Bromoacetyl-D-arginine	Glutamate
	Bromoacetyl-β-aminobenzyl- succinate	Methionine
α-Chymotrypsin	Tosyl-L-phenylalanine Chloromethyl-ketone (TPCK)	Histidine-57
	Glycidol phenyl-ether	Methionine-192
	Phenylmethansulphonyl fluoride (PMSF)	Serine-195
Formylglycinamide-ribotide amidotransferase	Azaserine	Cysteine
Fumarase	Bromomesaconate	Methionine Histidine
β-Galactosidase	N-Bromoacetyl-β-D-galactosylamine	Methionine
20-β-Hydroxysteroid dehydrogenase	Cortisone 21-iodoacetate	Histidine
Lactate dehydrogenase	3-Bromoacetyl pyridine	Cysteine, histidine
Lysozyme	2'3'-Epoxypropy-β-D-(N-acetyl glucosamine)$_2$	Aspartate 52
Methionyl-tRNA synthetase	p-Nitrophenyl-carbamyl-methionyl-tRNA	Lysine
RNA polymerase	5-Formyl-uridine-5'-triphosphate	Lysine
Staphylococcal nuclease	3'(N-Bromoacetyl-p-amino phenylphosphonyl) deoxy- thymidine-5'-phosphate	(Lysine -48 (Lysine -49 (Tyrosine -115
Triose phosphate isomerase	Glycidol phosphate	Glutamate

In the case of DIPF, the electrophilic phosphorus atom reacts with the nucleophilic hydroxyl group of the active-site serine residue, eliminating a fluoride ion and forming a stable DFP-enzymes. This is similar in some respects to the *acyl enzyme* intermediate formed in the normal hydrolytic reactions of these enzymes., Figure 9.1

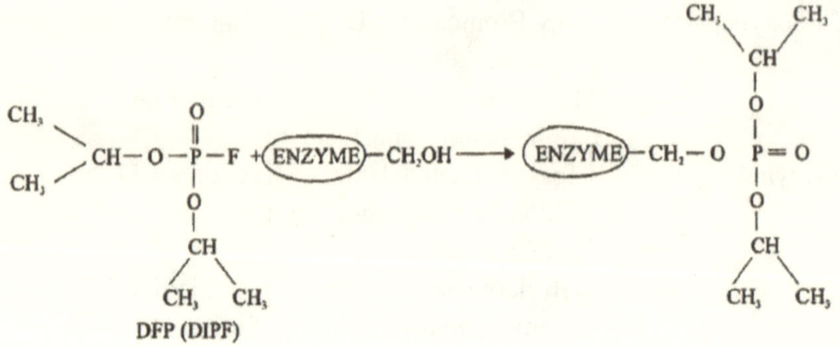

$$\text{(CH}_3\text{)}_2\text{CH}-\text{O}-\overset{\text{O}}{\underset{\text{O}-\text{CH(CH}_3\text{)}_2}{\overset{\|}{\text{P}}}}-\text{F} + \text{ENZYME}-\text{CH}_2\text{OH} \longrightarrow \text{ENZYME}-\text{CH}_2-\text{O}-\overset{\text{O}-\text{CH(CH}_3\text{)}_2}{\underset{\text{O}-\text{CH(CH}_3\text{)}_2}{\overset{\|}{\text{P}}}}=\text{O}$$

DFP (DIPF)

Figure 9.1: *Reactivity of the Diisopropylfluorophosphate (DIPF) with serine protease*

Certain aryl and alkylsulfonyl halides e.g. phenylmethanesulfonyl fluoride (PMSF) react with the active site serine residues of these same enzymes. Like the reaction with DIPF, these appear to result from some resemblances of these compounds to substrate of these enzymes. The greater the apparent resemblance to substrates, the greater the effectiveness.

9.4 AFFINITY LABELS

These possess substrate-like features. They take advantage of the normal enzyme-substrate interactions to ensure that large local concentration of the reagent (label) exists at the active site of the enzyme. The reactivity depends upon the ability of a reactive group in the affinity label to form a stable linkage to the enzyme. Thus, the reactive α-halocarbonyl in synthetic substrates (TLCK) group like the more familiar bromo-α-iodoacetate can react with several different nucleophilic groups found in the active site of several enzymes. So, TPCK (β(-toluene sulphonyl phenylalanine chloromethyl ketone) and TLCK (toluene sulphonyllysine chloromethyl ketone) are specific affinity labels for chymotrypsin and trypsin respectively. They are highly specific for the alkylation of histidine residues in the active centre of these enzymes. Affinity labels have been employed to determine residues in antibody combining sites. Some examples of affinity labels are listed in Table 9.3.

9.5 CROSS-LINKING REAGENTS

These are also called bi-functional reagents. They are reagents with two reactive groups, and they are useful for the following applications.

(i) Introduction of both inter-and intra-molecular cross-links into proteins
(ii) Preparation of cross-linked models for study of protein-protein interactions.
(iii) Serve as probes for determining distances between reactive groups in proteins.

The use of bi-functional reagents can be considered in terms of the two types of derivatives that can be formed; viz intra-molecular and intermolecular products

(a) The intra-molecular cross-linkages are used to stabilise the tertiary structure of proteins and to determine intramolecular distances between groups. The latter is accomplished by determining the particular amino acid residues linked by the two "heads" of individual bifunctional reagents. By using several reagents or by varying the distance between the two "heads" with several homologous reagents, it is possible to determine relative distances between several groups.

(b) The intermolecular cross-linkages may join molecules of the same kind in different ways. The products can be used, thus,

(i) for the study of protein-protein interactions, in high molecular weights analogs of one or both of the component proteins; or as substrates combining the desirable attributes of both components into one molecule;

(ii) to join biologically active molecules to insoluble carriers or to link adjacent subunits in naturally occurring subunit proteins as a means to determine their geometrical arrangement.

For example, dimethyl suberimidate has been used to study the subunit structure of several oligomeric proteins. This method appears capable of revealing some details of structure and reactivity of oligomeric proteins.

CHAPTER TEN

Regulation Of Enzyme Activity

10.0 GENERAL CONSIDERATION

The living cell seldom either synthesizes or degrades more material than is necessary for normal metabolism and growth. The regulation of cellular metabolism is concerned primarily with modulation of the key reactions that determine the fluxes of metabolites throughout the various pathways. Thus the control ultimately involves the regulation of enzyme activity. Broadly, enzymes can be regulated in two ways: genetic control and direct control of catalysis. Some of the regulatory mechanisms are illustrated in Figure 10.1

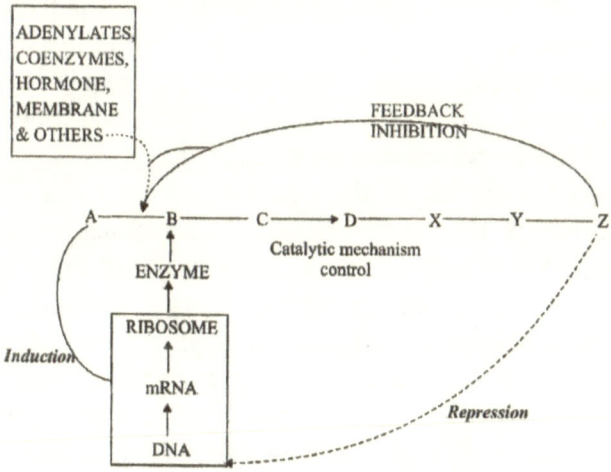

Figure 10.1: *Schematic representation of mechanisms for the regulation of enzyme activity*

(i) Genetic Control

The concentration of enzyme is determined by the rate of its synthesis and by the rate of its destruction. It is primarily determined by the rate of specific gene expression. In microorganisms, as well as in a few mammals, the addition of a substrate has been found to induce the synthesis of an enzyme which reacts with this particular substrate, conversely some compounds can cause the repression of enzyme synthesis. Thus, in catabolic pathways, two sets of enzymes exist; the *constitute enzymes* which are independent of substrate and *inducible enzymes* which are not normally present unless their immediate substrate or suitable derivatives thereof are present.

The substrate-induced synthesis of catabolic enzymes is sometimes repressed when the carbon and energy requirements for growth are amply supplied by a different catabolic pathway process. The mechanism of catabolic repression is not yet well established. In general, both induction and repression of enzyme synthesis act at the genetic level. The biochemical and genetic hypothesis involved have been extensively reviewed by Umbarger (1962) and Atkinson (1966).

(ii) Direct Control

The direct control of enzyme activity can occur through the catalytic mechanism itself or through a coupling of the catalytic mechanism with other processes. In the former case, the catalytic rate is dependent on the substrate concentration. As the substrate concentration increases, the reaction rate increases until a limiting value is reached; moreover, as the products accumulate, the reaction rate decreases (Michaelis-Menten kinetics). For many enzymes, coenzymes are necessary for catalysis. Since small amounts of coenzymes exist in the cell relative to the number of enzymatic reactions in which they are involved, the concentrations of these coenzymes could have a control function. Normally, the binding of substrate to enzyme follows a hyperbolic isotherm, but in enzymes with multiple subunits, the binding isotherm becomes sigmoidal owing to the effect of subunit interactions on substrate binding. (Figure 10.2).

This sigmoid binding curve has a region where the reaction rate is much more sensitive to the substrate concentration than is the case for a hyperbolic isotherm; therefore the rate of the enzymatic reaction can be closely regulated by the concentration of the substrate. The control of enzyme activity by coupling with other processes usually implies regulation by ligands which do not participate in the catalytic process, and in fact are often structurally unrelated to the substrate.

The major types of regulatory mechanisms of this category are enumerated below:

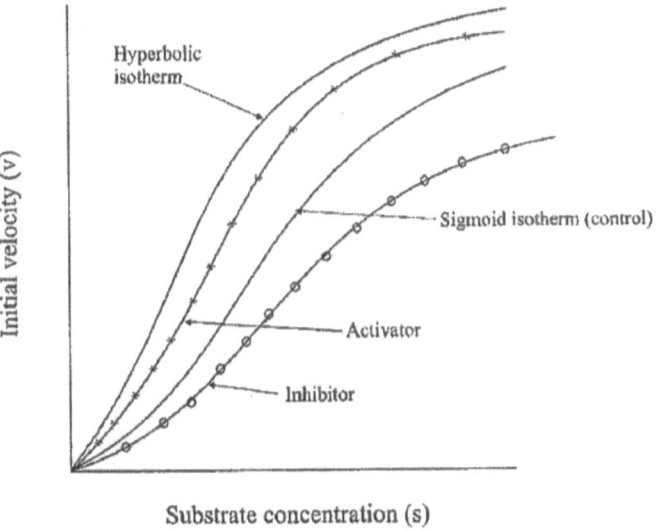

Figure 10.2: *Hyperbolic and sigmoid binding isotherms in direct control of enzyme activity*

10.1 TYPES OF REGULATORY MECHANISMS

(a) Feedback Inhibition

The regulatory ligand is the end product of a metabolic pathway, which can shut off its own formation by inhibiting the activity of one of the early enzymes on its own synthetic pathway. So, the end product usually exerts a restraining action through inhibition of the enzyme that catalyses the first step (committed step) in the biosynthetic pathway. (Scheme I). For example, threonine deaminase, the first enzyme in the biosynthetic pathway for isoleucine in *E. coli* is strongly inhibited by isoleucine even though isoleucine is not the substrate but end-product of the biosynthetic pathway.

Generally, the amino acid biosynthesis is regulated by feedback inhibition. The rate of synthesis of amino acids depends mainly on their enzymatic activities.

The final product of the pathway (z) often inhibits the enzyme that catalysed the committed step (A → B). This kind of control is essential for the conservation of building blocks and metabolic energy, Scheme 1.

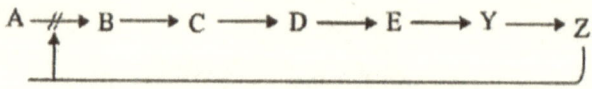

Scheme I: *Linear metabolic pathway*

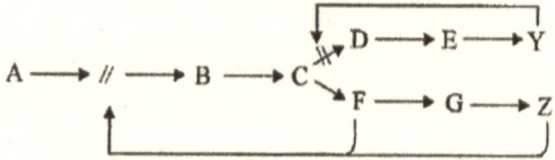

Scheme II: *Branched metabolic pathway*

Several intricate control mechanisms have been found in branched biosynthetic pathway. (Scheme II). These include sequential feedback control, enzyme multiplicity, concerted feedback control and cumulative feedback control. These various types of control will be discussed briefly:

(i) Sequential Feedback control

In this case, the first common step (A → B) is not inhibited directly by Y and Z, rather, three final products inhibit the reactions leading away from the point of branching. Y inhibits C → D step and Z inhibits the C → F step (Figure 10.3).

In turn high levels of C inhibits the A → B step. Thus the first common reaction is blocked only if both final products are present in excess.

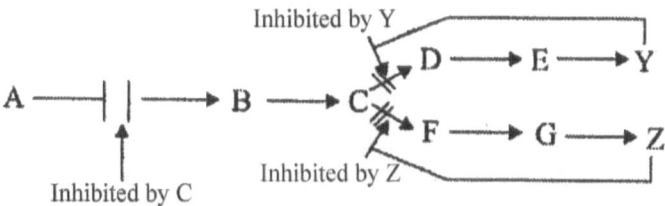

Figure 10.3: *Sequential Feedback Control*

Sequential feedback control is used to regulate the synthesis of aromatic amino acids in *Bacillus subtilis*.

(ii) Enzymes Multiplicity

The distinguishing feature of this mechanism is that the first common step (A → B) is catalysed by two different enzymes. One of them is inhibited by Y and the other by Z. Thus, both Y and Z must be present at high level to prevent the conversion of A to B completely. The other aspect of this control process is like that found in the sequential feedback control, Y inhibits the C → D step and Z inhibits C → F step, Figure 10.4.

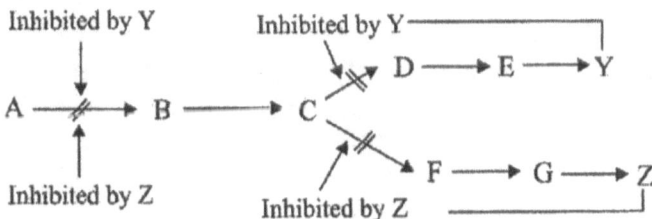

Figure 10.4: *Scheme for Enzyme multiplicity (feedback Inhibition)*

(iii) Concerted Feedback Control

The first common step (A → B) is inhibited only if high levels of Y and Z are simultaneously present. A high level of either product alone does not inhibit the A → B step. As in the control scheme discussed in (ii), Y inhibits the C → D step and Z inhibits the C → F step. (Figure: 10.5)

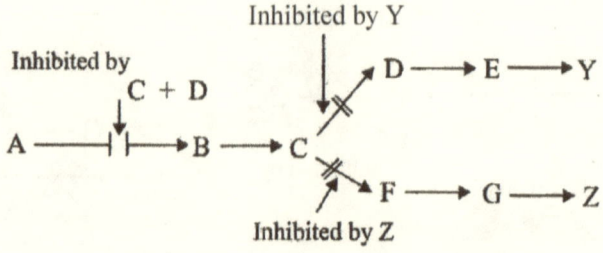

Figure 10.5: *Scheme for concerted feedback inhibition*

(iv) Cummulative Feedback Control

The first common step (A → B) is partially inhibited by each of the final products. Each final product acts independently of the others.

The regulation of the activity of glutamine synthetase in *E. coli* is a good example of cumulative feedback inhibition. Glutamine is synthesized from glutamate, NH_4^+ and ATP. The amide group of glutamine is a source of nitrogen in the biosynthesis of a variety of compounds such as tryptophan, histidine, carbamyl phosphate, CTP, and AMP. Glutamine synthetase is cumulatively inhibited by each of these final products of glutamine metabolism, and also by alanine and glycine. There seems to be specific binding sites for each of these inhibitors. The enzymatic activity of glutamine synthetase is almost completely switched off when all eight final products are bound to the enzyme.

(b) Precursor Activation

The regulatory ligand is the first metabolite of a pathway which activates the last enzyme of the sequence. For example, mammalian glycogen synthetase is activated by glucose 6-phosphate, a precursor of glycogen.

(c) Polymerization-Depolymerization

The association/dissociation reactions of a protein, for instance, multi- subunit enzymes or multi-enzyme complexes as triggered by changes in protein concentration or ligand binding can alter the enzyme activity. Such reactions may be either rapid, or slow and can lead to sigmoid binding of substrates.

(d) Energy-Link Control

The regulatory ligands are adenylates or other purine or pyrimidine nucleotides that may serve as indicators of the energy state of the cell. Energy in the cell is generated in the form of adenosine triphosphate (ATP) which is utilised in biosynthetic pathways, with the production of adenosine diphosphate (ADP) and monophosphates (AMP). The enzymatic reactions involved in energy generation are activation by ADP or AMP when the energy supply is low, and inhibited by ATP when the energy supply is high.

(e) Hormone Control

The regulatory ligand is a hormone which often regulates metabolism through a complex mechanism. For example, it can regulate the activity of adenyl cyclase, and the cyclic AMP produced regulates many metabolic processes.

(f) Covalent Modification

This type of control may involve phosphorylation/dephosphorylation process. In the synthesis and degradation of glycogen, for example, interconversions of phosphorylase b and a are catalysed by the enzyme phosphorylase kinase which requires magnesium ion ATP (phosphorylation) and phosphorylase phosphatase, (dephosphorylating enzyme).

Also, the activity of glutamine synthetase is regulated in part by the covalent attachment of an AMP unit to the hydroxyl group of a specific tyrosine residue in each subunit. This adenylylated enzyme is more susceptible to cumulative feedback inhibition than the deadenylylated form. The attachment of AMP to the enzyme is catalysed by *adenylyl transferase*. The AMP unit can be hydrolysed off the adenylated enzyme by deadenylyating enzyme. Glutamine activates adenylyl transferase and inhibits the deadenylylating enzyme.

10.2 MOLECULAR MECHANISMS OF ALLOSTERIC CONTROL

Several models have been postulated to explain non-linear Michaelis-Menten kinetics exhibited by allosteric enzymes. The most important ones are those due to Monod and co-workers (MWC); Koshland, Nemethy and Filmer (KNF) and that of Eigen and co-workers (EIG).

Some features are common to all the three models.

(i) Allosteric enzymes are assumed to be oligomers (small polymers) of identical subunits. (It is possible, however, to modify the models to include more than one type of subunit). A subunit may or may not be a single polypeptide chain.

(ii) There are multiple catalytic and regulatory binding sites on the subunits.

(iii) The change from active to inactive forms involves non-covalent forces and results in alteration of the quaternary structure of the enzyme. Changes in the subunits (tertiary) conformation also generally occur.

10.2.1 Special Features of the Molecular Models for Allosteric Control

(a) Monod, Wyman & Chargeux Model (MWC)

(i) There are two conformations, designated R and T, of an allosteric enzyme. These differ in tertiary and quaternary structure; in their affinities for substrates and for positive and negative allosteric effectors; and in catalytic activity. (Figure: 10.6).

(ii) All binding sites in a particular conformation; (R or T) are completely identical. This means that the only differences in affinity that can be observed are between R enzyme molecules and T enzyme molecules. On a given enzyme molecule, the binding of one substrate molecule does not affect the ease of binding of a second substrate molecule of the same type. (Figure: 10.6).

(iii) In a given enzyme molecule, all subunits are either in the R-form or the T-form. There are no mixtures of R- and T-subunits in the same enzyme molecule.

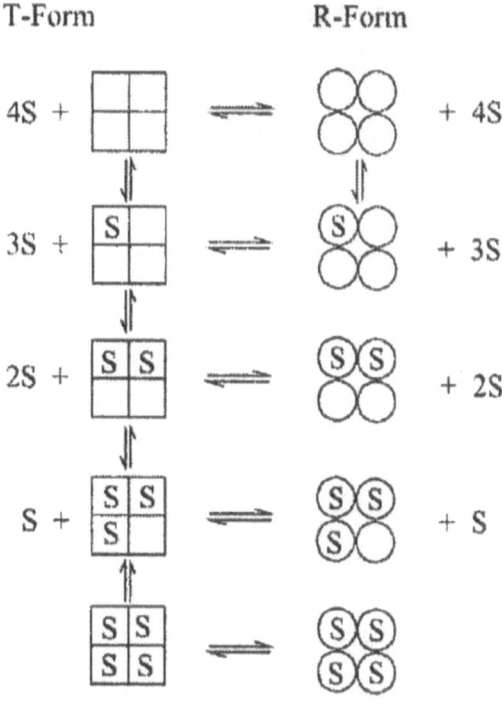

(where S is a substrate or effector molecule)

Figure 10.6: *Schematical Representation of Conformation States (MWC Model for the binding of ligands to a tetra- meric protein)*

With no ligand bound, the R- and T-forms are in equilibrium, with one form frequently predominating. As soon as a substrate (or effector) molecule binds, the enzyme molecule is "committed" to the form which it had when binding occurred. It cannot change form until all effector, substrate, or product molecules dissociate from it. (For example, the interconversion of S cannot occur directly). The binding of substrate or effector does not cause the conformational change.

Koshland, Nemethy and Filmer Model (KNF)

(i) In the absence of substrate or allosteric effectors, the enzyme exists in only one conformation. Figure: 10.7.
(ii) The binding of the substrate or effector to one of the subunits, causes that subunit to change conformation. This is popularly referred to as the induced-fit hypothesis.
(iii) The basis for co-operativity is the difference in interaction between subunits having substrate bound and those without substrate. That is, there is a difference circle-circle, circle-square, and square-square interactions as shown in Figure: 10.7.

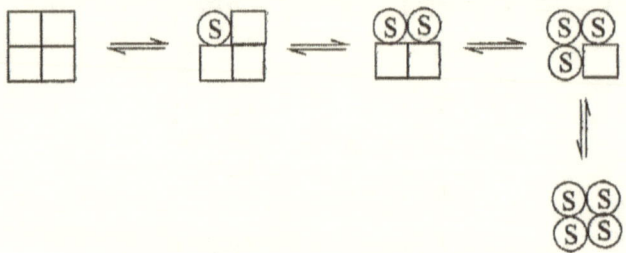

Figure 10.7: *Schematic representation of the (KNF model) conformation states - KNF model for the binding of ligands to a tetrameric protein*

REVIEW QUESTIONS (*Enzyme Catalysis, Mechanisms and Regulation*)

1. Discuss three approaches by which you can establish the active site of an enzyme.
2. Write notes on:

    (i) Nucleophilic Catalysis
    (ii) Enzyme Specificity
    (iii) Acid – base catalysis
    (iv) Metal – ion catalysis
    (v) Cross-linking reagents

ESSENTIALS OF ENZYMOLOGY 179

3. Discuss briefly, the "group specific" reagents, stating concisely the practical use of four of these in the elucidation of the active site of enzymes.

4. State two reagents that are specifically selective for the identification of the following amino acids in the active site of enzymes:

> Cysteine   Tyrosine
> Histidine   Lysine
> Tryptophan   Serine

Enumerate three methods by which these residues can be identified at the active centre

5. Discuss briefly the major regulatory mechanisms of enzyme activity.

6. Write a comprehensive essay on the mechanisms of enzyme regulation in intermediary metabolism.

7. Discuss briefly the allosteric control of enzyme activity.

8. Give a critical review of the suggested models of allosteric control of enzyme activity. State the THREE techniques for elucidating them.

9. Compare and contrast the features of the two outstanding molecular models advanced for the mechanism of allosteric control of enzyme activity.

10. Describe, giving relevant experimental evidences, in support of the proposed mechanism of action of either the Serine Proteases or Lysozyme.

11. Write concisely on the mechanism of action of the following:

    (i) Serine Proteases
    (ii) Dehydrogenases
    (iii) Lysozyme

REFERENCES

A. MOLECULAR BASIS FOR ENZYME REGULATION

1. D.E. Arkinson (1966). *Ann. Rev. Biochem.* 35, 85
2. E.R. Stadtman (1966). *Adv. Enzymology* 28, 41
3. D.E. Koshland, Jr. (1958). *P.N. A.S.* (U.S) 44, 98
4. D.E. Koshland, Jr (1968). & K.E. Neet - *Ann. Rev. Biochem* 37, 359
5. J.P Chargeux, - Cold Spring Harbor Sym. *Quant.Biol.* 26, 497
6. Conway and Koshland, Jr, (1968). *Biochemistry* 7, 4011
7. Cornish - Bowden & Koshland, (1970). *Biochemistry* 9, 3325

B. MECHANISM OF ENZYME REGULATION

1. Hegeman, G.D. (1966). *J. Bacterial,* 91, 319
2. Pallroni, N.J. & Stainer (1964). *J. Gen. Microbiol.* 35, 319
3. Ginsburg, A. (1969). *Biochemistry* 8, 1726
4. Gerhardt, J.G. & Schachman, (1965). *Biochemistry* 4, 1054
5. Monod et al. (1965). *Journal of Molecular Biology* 12, 88
6. Krebs, E.G. et al. (1958). *J. Biological Chem.* 231, 73
7. Shapiro, B.M. et al. (1967). *Proc. Natl. Acad. Sci.* (U.S) 58, 642
8. Shapiro, B.M. (1969). *Biochemistry* 8, 659
9. Walsh, D.A. *et al.* (1968). *J. Biol. Chem.* 243, 3763
10. Larner, J. (1967). *Ann. N.Y. Acad. Sci.* 29, 192
11. Koshland, Nemethy Filmer (1966). *Biochemistry,* 5, 365

PART IV

Applications Of Enzymology

CHAPTER ELEVEN

Enzymes In Clinical Diagnosis

11.0 INTRODUCTION

Enzymes have been known to exist in the human body for more than 80 years. The bulk of our knowledge and its clinical applications have come about only during the past 20 years, since Karmen demonstrated that raised aminotransferase levels accompanied mycocardial infraction. Previously, laboratory determinations of enzymic activity had accounted for a mere 3.5% of all examinations, and only a few enzymes had been studied. Today, 15-20% laboratory examinations are on the determination of enzyme activity and 15-18% different enzymes are examined routinely.

Enzymes are mostly contained in cells and their component parts. Furthermore, enzymes systems exhibit regular formations, especially within the cell, and these formations represent metabolic segments. The enzyme formation within an entire organ is also of prime importance, for example, the enzymes within the liver cells show different levels of activity in different parts of the hepatic lobule.

11.1 ENZYMES IN BLOOD PLASMA

The enzymes in blood plasma have been classified by Butcher into 3 main categories depending on their biological function and source (Table 11.1).

These include:

(i) **Plasma Specific Enzymes**

In this category,we have the blood clotting enzymes, cholinesterase, plasminogen. These enzymes have specific roles in blood.

(ii) **Secreted Enzymes**

In this group, we have most enzymes of pancreatic origin. These enzymes do not contribute to plasma function and are often catalytically ineffective through combination with the specific plasma inhibitors, for example, α-antitrypsin. Other enzymes in the group are prostate acid phosphatase.

(iii) **Cellular Enzymes**

In this group are the enzymes of tissue metabolism (catabolic enzymes) and those of key metabolic pathways. These include aldolase, α-glycerophosphate dehydrogenase, lactate dehydrogenase, malate dehydrogenase, amino-transferases. Also included in the group are the organ-specific enzymes; urea cycle enzymes; alkaline phosphatase; glucose-6-phosphatase.

Table 11.1: *Classification of enzymes in blood*

	Group	Examples
(i)	Plasma specific enzymes	Prothrombin, Plasminogen, Ceruloplasmin, Lipoprotein Lipase, Pseudo-cholinesterase
(ii)	Secreted enzymes	Pancreatic, parotid a-amylase, prostatic phosphatase, pepsinogen
(iii)	Cellular enzymes	Lactate dehydrogenase, malate dehydrogenase, a-glycerophosphate dehydrogenase
	(a) Enzymes of tissue metabolism and Key-metabolic pathways	
	(b) Organ-specific enzymes	Urea cycle enzymes, Sorbitol dehydrogenase Glucose-6-phosphatase, Bone alkaline phosphatase

11.2 FACTORS WHICH CONTROL ENZYME LEVELS IN BLOOD PLASMA

The enzyme levels in blood plasma depend on three main factors, namely:

(i) the turnover and proliferation of cells with access to the blood plasma.
(ii) the total enzymes complement.
(iii) the intracellular enzymes distribution.

The tissue dependent level of activity in the blood is a function of two vectors; thus (a) the flux of extrication from the cells and (b) the fluxes of inactivation, degradation and elimination from the plasma, These vectors depend on the state of health of the individual. The constant low level of enzymes is the result of normal cell turnover which support the concept of co-ordinated process regulating cell turnover and metabolism. For instance, the red blood cells with average turnover of 5×10^5 has increased turnover in hemolytic anaemia, hence causing the associated plasma enzyme activities to be increased.

In the serum of healthy individual, studies of enzyme activities particularly transaminases show a consistent, virtually constant pattern of activity, hence, it suggests the existence of a regulatory process in the body. However, an increase of enzyme activity in serum is due to damage to the cells of the organ. Studies on experimental animals have shown that there is a good correlation between the increase in activity of individual enzymes in serum and the dose of a toxin or concentration of virulence of an injected virus or the size of the supply of a ligated vessel. Clinical studies have also shown good correlation between the severity of the disease and the extent of the enzyme changes in serum. For instance, the lactate dehydrogenase (LDH) isoenzyme patterns of red blood cells and blood plasma are different.

Generally, enzymes are released from hepatocytes, osteoblasts, spleen, and endothelial cells, with direct access to the blood. The alteration in blood plasma enzymes levels can be brought about through exercise, haemo-concentration, hormonal changes, nutritional imbalances. Moreover, when anabolic-catabolic equilibrium which maintains energy balance is perturbed by anoxia, hypoglycemia or starvation, then the intracellular osmolality rise, membrane permeability increase and enzyme leakage will occur.

The suggested mechanisms for the release of intracellular enzymes from tissues damaged by a pathological process is depicted below, Figure 11.1

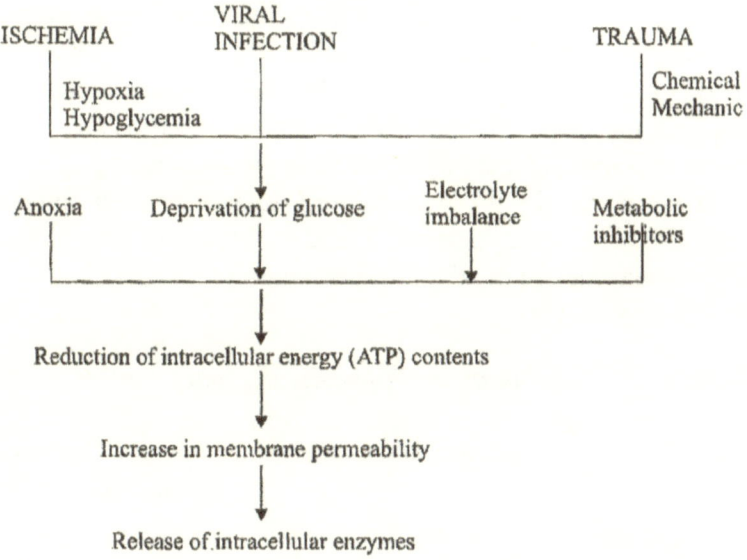

Figure 11.1: *Postulated mechanisms for the release of intracellular enzymes from tissues damaged by a pathological process.*

11.3 CLINICAL SIGNIFICANCE OF ENZYME ANALYSIS

The activities of individual enzymes in the blood are determined when it is expected that the levels will be raised as a result of release from the tissues. This occurs when the cell membrane has been modified in some way that it loses its selectivity and become permeable to proteins. The blockage of biological oxidative processes or obstruction of the transformation of oxidative energy to chemical binding energy also leads to the release of enzymes into the blood plasma.

The urinary excretion of enzymes depends on the renal function so that this introduces a complicating factor in the calculation of enzyme activity.

In cerebrospinal fluid, enzyme activity may be elevated in the presence of lesions of the central nervous systems of the blood-brain barrier. Enzyme activity in the tissues, most especially from the organs - liver, kidneys, and the muscles is possible nowadays to the availability of a great variety of biopsy techniques. The examination of liver tissue helps both the assessment of liver function and also in the diagnosis of congenital metabolic and enzyme defects. Other tissues that may also be examined include bone, prostate, tumour, collagen, and ovary. Changes in the activity of specific enzymes on their deficiency could aid to elucidate a variety of both congenital and acquired metabolic defects. The distribution of diagnostically important enzymes in medicine is presented in Table 11.2.

Table 11.2: *Distribution of diagnostically important enzymes*

Enzyme	Principal Source	Principal Clinical Application
Acid phosphatase	Prostate, Erythrocytes	Carcinoma of prostate
Alanine aminotransferase, (ALT)	Liver, skeletal muscle, heart	Muscle disease
Amylase	Salivary glands, pancrease, ovaries	Pancreatic diseases
Alkaline phosphatase	Liver, bone, intestinal mucosa placenta, kidney	Bone disease Hepato-biliary disease
Cholinesterase	Liver	Hepatic parenchyma Disease
Aspartate Aminotransferase, (AST)	Liver, skeletal, muscle, heart, Kidney, erythrocytes	Myocardial infraction Muscle disease Hepatic disease
γ-glutamyltransferase	Liver, kidney	Hepatobiliary disease
Lactate dehydrogenase	Heart, liver, skeletal muscle Platelets, lymph nodes	Myocardial infraction Hepatic disease
5'Nucleotidase	Hepatobiliary tract	Hepatobiliary disease
Trypsinogen	Pancreas	Pancreatic disease

Examination of groups of enzymes produces so called enzyme spectra that ease the finer points of differential diagnosis, for example, in liver disease. (Example: AST, ALS, spectra ALP and type of hepatopathy).

Enzyme activities can be determined in sperm, aspirates, ascitic fluid, synovial fluid and other biological fluids. The ability to cultivate fibroblasts and to examine them for certain enzymic defects means that amniotic fluid obtained in the third month of pregnancy can now be used to detect a heterozygote suffering form a congenital metabolic defect.

11.4 CLINICAL APPLICATIONS

(i) Bone Disease

Alkaline phosphatase (ALP) participates in the calcification of bone, therefore its activity is higher in children than in adults. The activity is raised to very high levels in patients with ricketts, osteomalacia, Paget's disease (osteitis deformans) osteoblastic Paget's sarcoma and metastatic carcinoma. In all these diseases, the high activity is of great diagnostic value. In bone disease, repeated checks of alkaline phosphatase activity are most important. The activity of the enzymes is also elevated in obstruction of the bile ducts.

Acid phosphatase, too, is present in the bone, and its activity can be moderately elevated but bone phsophatase can be differentiated from prostatic phosphatase.

(ii) Gastrointestinal Disease

High levels of serum pepsinogen are often found in peptic ulcer of the stomach, though they may be normal or low. The levels are always low in gastric carcinoma. Roughly, half of the patients with duodenal ulcer have markedly raised levels. Decrease serum pepsinogen levels are always found in pernicious anemia. Trypsin estimation in duodenal juice can serve as an indicator of pancreatic function, but a low result does not always prove pancreatic insufficiency.

(iii) Liver Disease

Liver function tests are based on a number of changes accompanying damage to the liver parenchyma. Consequently, disturbances appear first in the diseases that effect the parenchyma form such as hepatitis. It is important to note that each individual test gives information solely about one component of liver function; therefore, several different types of tests must be performed to obtain a reliable assessment of liver function.

The enzyme spectra that assist in the assessment of the type and degree of hepatic lesion include tests for the activities of asparatate (AST) and alanine (ALT) aminotransferases; leucine aminotransferate (LAS), ornithine carbomyltransferase (OCT), glutamate dehydrogenase (GMD), alkaline phosphatase (ALP) and cholinesterase (CHS). Gamma-glutamyltransferase (γ-GT), is often raised, but it is especially reactive to chronic hard consumption of alcohol. In infectious mononucleosis, the serum enzyme activities are elevated in a similar manner to liver disease.

(iv) Myocardial Infraction

Enzyme tests are often useful in myocardial infraction. The most important tests are those for the serum levels of Creatine kinase and its MB isoenzymes, aspartate aminotransferase, lactate dehydrogenase and its LDH isoenzymes. Their peak levels appear on about the second day after the onset of pain and on the 5th to 6th day, the levels return to normal. In patients suffering from *angina pectoris,* the serum enzyme levels as a rule lie within normal limits or rise only insignificantly.

(v) Prostatic Disease

The prostate is the organ richest in acid phosphatase. The prostatic variety of the enzyme posed several characteristic properties, allowing it to be differentiated from acid phosphatases originating form other cells or tissues, such as erythrocytes or bone. An elevation of prostatic carcinoma reflects as a rule, the presence of metastatic prostatic carcinoma. During the initial stages before *metastasizing occurs,* the serum acid phosphatase is usually elevated in only a quarter of the patients, since the enzyme enters the urinary tract.

CHAPTER TWELVE

Enzyme Biotechnology

12.0 INTRODUCTION

Biotechnology is a set of powerful tools that employ living organisms (or parts of organism) to make or modify product, improve plant or animal or development of microorganisms for specific uses. Examples of the "new biotechnology" include the industrial use of recombinant DNA, cell fusion, novel bioprocess techniques and bioremediation.

In the area of biocatalysis, the nature's catalysts enzymes, whose function is highly selective do accelerate the rate of chemical reactions in biological systems. Also, they can limit chemical reactivity towards a particular substrate and this limit chemical conversion to a single desired product. The ability to mimic the selectivity and rate enhancing properties of enzymes are of substantial benefits in reducing economic and environmental costs.

Protein engineering, chemical modifications, and recombinant monoclonal antibody technology are areas of research in the development and application of new enzymes of industrial importance. They also generate catalysts that exhibit the useful characteristics of naturally occurring enzymes. In particular, enzyme engineering has played significant roles in the development of new biotechnological firms' works that include:

1.1 production of value-added products for the drug and food industries;
1.2 marketing a patented enzyme for the drugs and chemical market;
1.3 marketing various biological synthesis capabilities for the agricultural and drug industries, and
1.4 the molecular modelling and development of research software.

At present, about 50 enzymes are used in industry (Table 12.1). Most of the industrial uses involve breaking down large molecules into simpler ones. Examples, include the proteases in laundry detergents and hydrolases in starch processing. Production of sweetness i.e.enhanced corn syrup by the enzyme glucose isomerase is noteworthy, an example of how a chemical transformation can be carried out on the industrial scale. Some examples of industrial enzymes are presented in Table 12.2.

12.1 INDUSTRIAL USES OF ENZYMES

12.1.1 Dairy

In the dairy industry, enzymes are essential for the production of cheese. Milk contains a group of proteins called caseins. One of the proteins, kappa-casein prevents milk from coagulation in the presence of calcium ions. The enzyme, renin, which has traditionally been obtained from the lining of calves' stomachs, breaks down casein into the smaller protein called para-casein. Once the kappa-casein is destroyed, coagulation occurs to form a soft curd that can be separated from the liquid form of the milk. The curd is the starting material of the production of cheese. The fluid remaining after the curd is separated is "whey". It contains among other components, proteins and non-sweet sugar, lactose.

The demand by the cheese industry for renin is very large, so substitutes for the calf product, microbial engineered product has been developed and is widely used. Nowadays, however, it produces cheese of slightly inferior quality because the microbial enzyme is harder to inactivate than the calf product when its action is no longer desired. Whey has in the past presented a disposal problem. However, current research has explored methods of using enzymes to convert whey into a material that can be used as an additive to foods. If it is treated with the enzyme, lactase, the lactose is broken into two sweet digestive sugars: glucose and galactose. The resulting sweet, protein-rich syrup can be added to certain food products, such as ice-cream.

12.1.2 Beverages

In the beverage industry, enzymes are used to chill-proof juices, wines and beer. Juices and wines contain a polysaccharide called pectin that is soluble at room temperature but, when cooled, may form a colloidal suspension that gives the liquid a cloudy appearance. To prevent the haze from forming, enzymes called pectinases are added to the juice or wine. The enzymes degrade the pectin to lower molecular weight and therefore more soluble, fragments that do not precipitate on cooling. The similar problem of haze formation occurs during beer manufacture which is caused by proteins and tannins rather than polysaccharides. To chill-proof beer, proteases such as pepsin or papain are added to break down the proteins and limit the formation "chillhaze" as it is called.

12.1.3 Confectionery

The confections are first made with solid centers that contain the enzyme, invertase. Over a period of three to four weeks, the invertase transforms the sucrose into a liquid mixture of fructose and glucose. In addition to being sweeter than sucrose, fructose has the advantage of retaining more moisture, so that it preserves and also prevents the sweets drying out and tasting stale.

Enzymes are also important in packaging foods. For example, the plastic wrapper used for cheese may be coated with two enzymes, glucose oxidase and peroxidase to prevent spoilage. Under the influence of the glucose oxidase, the oxygen reacts instead with the glucose in the plastic wrapper to form gluconic acid and hydrogen peroxidase which is converted to water by peroxidase. Glucose oxidase is often added to mayonnaise to prevent spoilage by oxidation. However, the amount of enzymes added in these applications is very small.

Table 12.1: *Important uses of enzymes*

INDUSTRY	APPLICATION	ENZYME	SOURCE
Analytical	Sugar determination	Glucose oxidase	Fungi
	Glycogen determination	Galactose oxidase	Fungi
		Glucoamylase	Fungi, plant
	Urea determination	Urease	Plant
	Uric acid determination	Lipoxygenase	Malt, fungi
		Amylase	Fungi
		Protease	Fungi
Baking and Milling	Bread Baking	Amylase	Malt, fungi
		Protease	fungi
		Lipoxygenase	Plant
Brewing	Mashing	Amylase	Malt, bacteria
	Chillproofing	Glucoamylase	Fungi
		Protease	fungi, Bacteria
		Papain	
		Bromelain	
		Pepsin,	
Carbonated Beverages	Oxygen removal	Glucose oxidase	Fungi
	Oxygen removal	Glucose oxidase	Fungi
Cereals	Precooked baby Foods	Amylase	Malt; fungi
		Amylase	Malt, fungi
	Breakfast foods	Protease	fungi, bacteria
	Condiments	Papain	
		Bromelain	
		Pepsin	
Chocolate, Cocoa coffee	Syrups	Amylase	Bacterial, fungi
	Coffee bean fermentation	Pectinase	Fungi
		Pectinase,	Fungi

	Coffee concentrates	Hemicellulase	Yeast
Confectionery, (candy)	Soft-centre candies and fondants Sugar recovery from scrap candy	Invertase Amylase	Bacteria, fungi
Dairy	Cheese production	Rennin	fungal, Animal
	Milk: Sterilization with Peroxide Modifying milk fats Lipase for flavour	Catalase	Liver, bacterial, Fungi
	Milk: prevention of Protease oxidized flavour		Pancreatin
	Milk, protein Hydrolyzation	Protease Papain Bromelain Pancreatin	Bacteria, fungi.

12.2 Medicinal Applications of Enzymes

A myriad of chemical reactions occurring in the body are catalyzed and controlled by enzymes. Enzymes mediate the digestion of food, build the components of cells, generate and respond to intracellular messengers such as hormones and the chemical neurotransmitter that carry nerve signals. Thus enzymes are valuable both for studying these complicated systems and for medical therapies.

Such therapeutic applications include the simple use of pancreatin (mixture of pancreatic enzymes) as digestive aid to people who are deficient in digestive enzymes as a result of genetic disorders, surgical removal of gall bladder or advancing age.

A more complex medical application involves the use of the enzyme *Heparinase* for controlling blood clotting. Patients who are undergoing kidney dialysis or certain forms of surgery or who have had heart attacks or strokes are often treated with a polysaccharide called heparin which acts to decrease the ability of the blood to clot. Heparinase selectively cuts heparin apart thereby destroying its activities.

Other therapeutic enzymes include Tissue Plasminogen Activator (TPA) which promotes the dissolution of the blood clots that form during heart attacks; Urokinase, Pro-urokinase and Streptokinase, which also have clot-dissolving activities. All of them do have therapeutic benefits for heart attack victims.

Table 12.2: *Some Examples of Industrial Enzymes: Their Sources & Uses*

ENZYME	SOURCE	USE
Alkaline proteases	Microorganisms	Detergents
Renin	Calf & Lamb Stomachs; Microbes	Cheese Production
Papain	Papaya	Meat: Beer, Leather industries, Textiles, pharmaceuticals; Digestive aid; dental; hygiene, Clarification of beer haze.
Bromelain	Pineapple	Meat: baking, pharmaceutical, Meat, beer, leather, pharmaceuticals industries
Ficin	Figs	Meat, beer, leather industries, pharmaceuticals
Pepsin	Hog stomach	Cereals; pharmaceuticals, feeds

Trypsin	Hog & Calf pancreas	Meat, pharmaceuticals
Amylase	Fungi; plants; Recombinant Organisms.	Hydrolysis of starch for ethanol production; detergents, milk, cheese, fruit-juices; digestive aids; dental hygiene
Invertase	Yeast	Invert-sugar production, confectionery, beverages.
Glucose isomerase	Microorganisms	Conversion of glucose to fructose in production of High-fructose corn syrup, soft drinks; also other beverages and foods.
Pectinases	Fungi, tomatoes	Hydrolysis of pectic substances for clarification of fruit juices, wine, coffee; cocoa industries.
Glucose oxidase	Microoganisms	Oxidation glucose to glucuronic acid; preservation of flavour & colour in eggs, and fruit juice.
p-amylase	Microbes	Production of maltose; Baked products; digestive aids,
Pullulanase	Microbes	Production of beer, maltose and glucose
Cellulase	Microbes	Ethanol production, Digestive aids
Urokinase	Urine	Treatment of thrombosis
Asparaginase	*Escherichia coli*	Antitumor agent
Lipases	Hog kidney; & Calf Pancreas	Hydrolysis of fat and fatty acid esters; detergents, chocolate, cheese; feed, digestive aids

Catalase & Lipoxidase	Liver	Breakdown of hydrogen peroxide, milk sterilization; production of cheese; bleaching agent in baking industry
Penicillin acylase	*Escherichia coli*	Production of 6-aminopenicillanic acid for synthesis of various P-lactam antibiotics

12.3 IMMOBILIZED ENZYMES

Introduction

The term "immobilised enzymes" can be defined as a system or preparation in which an enzyme is confined or localized in a relatively defined region or space. The enzyme can be attached by one of several mechanisms to a supporting solid surface or simply physically confined within a surrounding solid or liquid barrier. The enzyme can be used continuously in flow processes or repetitively in batch contacts as long as the enzyme preparation is active.

12.3.1 Historical Perspectives

Nelson and Griffin (1916) prepared the first immobilized enzyme and the immunologists made the first use of this methodology in the isolation of antibodies. They adsorbed and later covalently bound antigens to solid supports for the isolation of specific antibodies.

The period, (1930 - 1950) witnessed the development of some important early techniques including the chemical modification of available carriers such as polystryrene and cellulose for the purpose of improving immunoadsorbent preparations. These were applied to enzyme immobilisation and a considerable number of carriers with varying degree of hydrophobicity were developed.

Subsequently, during the period, (1960 - 1970), research was parallel in three major frontiers:

(i) the pre-design of carriers in order to achieve optimal binding and enzyme stability:
(ii) the development of milder and more general techniques of immobilization as an alternative to covalent methods;
(iii) the study of immobilised enzymes in continuous flow-packed bed and continuous stirred tank reactors.

The period, (1970 - 1975) witnessed the development of enzyme technology - (enzyme engineering). This discipline emerged from the principles of enzymology and chemical engineering techniques, see Figure 12.1.

12.4 CLASSIFICATION

The immobilised enzymes can be classified in several ways. These include:

(a) type of interactions responsible for immobilisation;
(b) the nature of support;
(c) the nature of the resulting complex and
(d) the type of reactions catalysed by the enzyme.

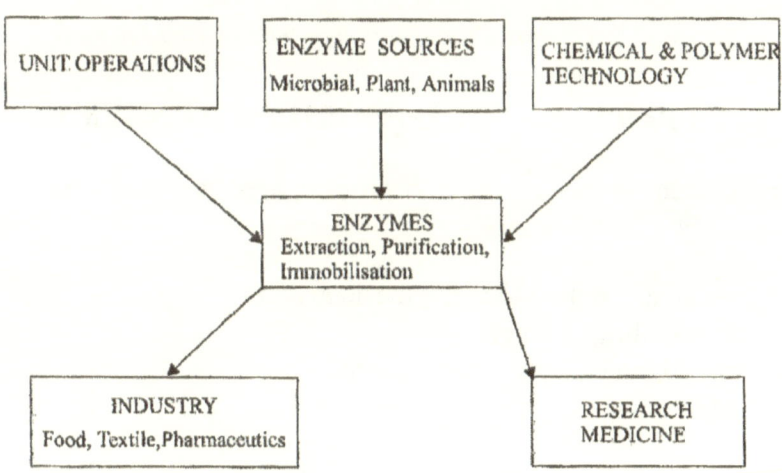

Figure 12.1: *Inter-Relationship of Major Areas of "Enzyme Engineering"*

Invariably, the classification based on (a) is most favoured; as enumerated either by chemical methods that depend on the formation of at least one covalent bond per molecule or physical methods which utilise non-covalent bond formation or simple entrapment. Thus, immobilised enzymes may be classified as either "entrapped" or "bound". The former group includes matrix-entrapped and microcapsulated enzymes whilst the latter includes adsorbed, covalent bound and cross-linked enzymes. The general classification of immobilised enzymes is depicted in Figure 12.2.

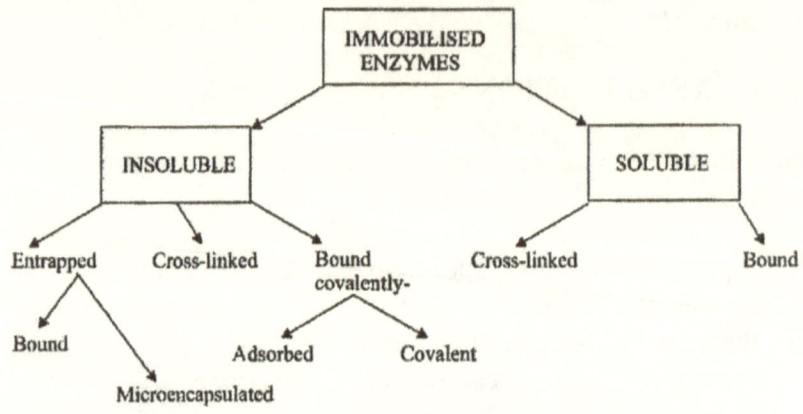

Figure 12.2: *General Classification of Immobilised Enzymes*

12.5 PREPARATION OF IMMOBILISED ENZYMES

Immobilised enzymes have been prepared by the following procedures:

(i)   covalent coupling to a polymeric matrix;
(ii) cross-linking methods;
(iii) adsorption on a polymeric matrix;
(iv) entrapment within a polymeric matrix.

So far, over 500 different enzymes have been immobilised and characterised in about 2,000 technical reports to date.

12.6 CRITERIA FOR CHOICE OF CARRIER AND IMMOBILIZATION

The 'best' choice of carrier depends considerably on the enzyme and on the type of application in which it is to be utilized. Similarly, characteristics can vary considerably for the same enzyme bound to different carriers or to a single carrier by different techniques. The important parameters for the characterization of immobilized enzymes include:

(i) **Activity Profile:** The expressed activities of immobilized enzymes are sensitive to environmental conditions such as substrate concentration, effector concentration, temperature, pH, ionic strength, etc.

(ii) **Bound Protein:** The amount of protein bound to the carrier is a better method of characterizing the effectiveness of a particular immobilization technique, since activity measurements are very sensitive to assay conditions.

(iii) **The Coupling Yield:** This is defined as:

$$\frac{\text{overall activity of insolubilized enzyme}}{\text{overall activity of the initial enzyme}} \times 100$$

predicts the efficacy of the immobilised enzyme.

(iv) **Stability of Carrier-Enzyme Complex**

The stability of an immobilised enzyme preparation can be characterized in several different ways. One approach is to determine the shelf-life or storage stability of the preparation by measuring the activity during regular intervals whilst stored wet or dry at specific environmental conditions. The much more valuable characterization is called operational stability of the system, which is determined by monitoring the activity of the immobilized enzyme during continuous use under environmental condition that the system will encounter in its ultimate application.

12.7 APPLICATIONS FOR IMMOBILIZED ENZYMES

The immobilized enzymes have been employed for various applications in the following areas: industry, medical, analytical and research. These have been listed below;

1. **Industrial**
   - production of high fructose corn syrup
   - production of L-aminoacids from the acyl-D-L-amino acids
   - production of semi-synthetic penicillin intermediates.
   - Cheese-whey lactose hydrolysis by bound β-galactosidase
   - beer-chill proofing
   - steroid transformations
   - removal of residual oxygen in various food products
   - production of drug metabolites
   - structural modification of Cephalosporin C.

2. **Analytical:**
   Manufacture of specific enzyme electrodes for the determination of specific metabolites, for example - glucose, urea, uric acid.

3. **Medical:**
   - analysis of metabolites in body fluids
   - treatment of hereditary enzyme defects
   - biochemical research
   - treatment of enzyme - sensitive disorders.

12.8 ENZYME BIOINFORMATICS

Bioinformatics is the term given to the collection, storage, communication, analysis and interpretation of biological data. The processing aspects are heavily dependent on the information in the databases, communicated by means of the Internet. The task used in bioinformatics concerns the creation and maintenance of biological information. The nucleic acids sequences (and the proteins sequences derived from them) comprises the majority of such databases.

The analysis of sequence information is known as Computational Biology and this involves.

(a) Find the genes in the DNA sequences of various organisms.
(b) Developing methods to predict the structure and or function of newly discovered proteins and structural RNA sequences.
(c) Classifying proteins sequences into families of related sequences and the development of proteins models.
(d) Aligning similar proteins and generating phylogenetic trees to examine evolutionary relationships.

Some application uses of bioinformation are listed below:

(i) Identification of specific amino residues in the active site of enzymes. For the Human glucocerebrosidase, thus, Glu 235 and Glu 340 were found to be putative acid / base catalyst and nucleophile respectively. This may help to better stand the molecular basis of Gaucher's disease, the human lysosomal disease resulting from the deficiency in glucocerebrosidase, (Fabrega et al, 2000).
(ii) Deduce the gene sequence and organisation of the highly homologous Drosophilia melanogaster orthologue of lucilia curprina chitin synthetase-like protein (LcCS-1) Tellan et al, 2000.
(iii) Indicate the presence of at least six carbonic anhydrates or the closely related genes in the genome of fruit fly, Droosophila melanogaster. (delpillar-Corena, M. 2002).
(iv) Identify and functionally express a UDP-D-glucuronate 4 - epimerase from Arabdopsis Plants. (Molhoj *et al,* 2004).
(v) Identify a number of genes in thermophilic viruses with potential use in biotechnology. (Blondal,.*et al.* 2003).

References

(i) Fabrega, S. Durand, P; Codogno, P, Bauvy C; Delomenia, C. Henrissat B, Martin, B, M. Makinney C. Ginn, E. I. Morno, J.P. and Lehn, P. (2000). Human glucocerebrosidase: Heterologous expression of active site munants in murine null cells." Glycobiology 10 (11) 1217 - 1224.

(ii) Tellan, R. L, Vuocolo, T; Johnson S. E; Jarmey J. and Peurson, R. D. (2000) "Insect Chitin Synthetase cDNA sequences, gene organisation and expression - Eur. J. Biochem. 267 (19) 6025 - 6043.

(iii) Rapisarda, V. A.; Chehin, R, N; De-las Rivas, J; Rodriguez - Montelongo, L; Farias, R. N; Massa, E. A. (2002) - "Evidence for Cu (I) thiolase ligation and prediction of a putative copper - binding site in the Escherichia Coli, NADH dehydrogenase - 2 - Arch. Biochem. Biophys. 405 (1) 87 - 94.

(iv) Del-Pillar Corena, M, Seron, T. J. Lehman; H. K. Ochrietor, J. D. Kohn, A. Tu-Chingkuang, Linser, P. J. (2002) Carbonic anhydrase in the midgnut of Larial Aedes aegypti: cloning, localization and inhibition. J. Expt. Bio. 205 (pt 50 591 - 602.

(v) Molhoj, M. Verma, R. and Reiter, W. D. (2004). The biosynthesis of D-Galactruronate in Plants: Functional cloning and characterisation of a membrane - anchored UDP - D-glucuronate 4-epimerase from Arabidopis - Plant Physiol, 135 (3). 1221 - 1230.

(vi) Blodal, T., Hjorleifdottir, S. H. Fridjonson, O. F; Aevarsoon, Smith A. V. Kristjansson, J. K. (2003) - Discovery and characterization of a thermostable bacteriophage RNA lipase hormologus to T_4 RNA Sigase 1. - (2003). Nucleic Acids Res. 31 (24) 7247 - 7254.

REVIEW QUESTIONS

1. Discuss the application of enzymes in medicine with special reference to diagnostic and therapeutic uses.
2. Describe the practical approaches involved in enzyme immobilization. What are the advantages and disadvantages of an immobilized enzyme system?

REFERENCES

Friedel, R, Diederichs, F. Lindena, J. (1979). "Release and extracellular turnover of intracellular enzymes". In: *Advances in Clinical Enzymology* Eds. Basel, Kargen. pp. 70-105.

Lee, T.H & Goldman (1986). "Serum assays in the diagnosis of acute myocardial infarction". *Ann. Intern. Med.* 105: 221-221.

Lott, J. A., Lu, C.T. (1991). "Lipase isoforms, and amylase isoenzymes. : Assay and application in the diagnosis of acute pancreatitis". *Clin. Chem.* 37: 361-368.

Oesterling, J.E. (1991). "Prostate specific antigen: A critical assessment of the most useful tumor marker for adenocarcinoma of the prostrate". *J. Urol.* 145 907-923

Raymond, F. Datta H, Moss, D.W. (1991). "Alkaline phosphate isoforms in bile and serum; and their generation from cells *in vitro*". *Biochim. Biophys.* Acta 1074, 217-222

Wu, A.H.B (1989). "Creatinc kinase isoforms in ischemic heart disease", *Clin. Chem.* 35, 7-13.

Jones M. G., Swaminathan R. (1990). "The clinical biochemistry of creatine kinase",. *J. Int. Fed. Clin. Chem.* 2. 108-114.

ENZYME BIOTECHNOLOGY

Bullock J.and Kristiansen B (Editors) (1987). *Basic Biotechnology.* Academic Press, London

Colon H.D and Walt D R. (1986). "Immobilization of Enzymes in Polymer supports". *J. Chem Educ.* 63 368-370

Kennedy J. F and White C. A. (1985). "Principles of Immobilization of Enzymes". In: *Handbook of Enzyme Biotechnology* (Edited by Wiseman A.) 2nd Edn. Pp. 147-207 Ellis Horwood Chichester

Maerz U and Wenck H (1989). "The industrial use of enzymes – some classrooms experiments". *Biotech. Educ.* 1. 23-27

Roig M. G., Esterez F. B. Velasco F. G. Ghais, N. I. and Silverio J. M. C (1986). "Methods for Immobilizing Enzymes". *Biochem. Educ.* 14 180-185

Suggestions for Further Reading:

Malik V. S. (1982). Biotechnology and where it is going - *Process Biochemistry* March/April 1982. pp 38-41

Malik, V. S. (1989) "Biotechnology – The Golden Age". In: *Advances in Applied Microbiology.* 34, 263- 305.

Grunwald, P. (1986). "Enzyme Technology.: A practical topic in basic chemical education". *J. Chem. Educ.* 63, 775 – 776

Kierstan, M. P. J. and Coughlan M. P. (1985) "Immobilization of cells and enzymes by gel entrapment". In: *Immobilised cells and Enzymes – A practical Approach* (Edited by Woodward J.) pp. 39-48 IRL Press, Oxford

APPENDIX

I. NOMENCLATURE & CLASSIFICATION OF ENZYMES

Key to Numbering and Classification of Enzymes

1. OXIDOREDUCTASES

1.1 Acting on the CH-OH group of donors
    1.1.1 With NAD^+ or $NADP^+$ as acceptor
    1.1.2 With a cytochrome as acceptor
    1.1.3 With oxygen as acceptor
    1.1.9 With other acceptors
1.2 Acting on the aldehyde or oxo group of donors
    1.2.1 With NAD^+ or $NADP^+$ as acceptor
    1.2.2 With a cytochrome as acceptor
    1.2.3 With oxygen as acceptor
    1.2.4 With a disulphide compound as acceptor
    1.2.7 With an iron-sulphur protein as acceptor
    1.2.9 With other acceptors
1.3 Action on the CH-CH group of donors
    1.3.1 With NAD^+ or $NADP^+$ as acceptor
    1.3.2 With a cytochrome as acceptor
    1.3.3 With oxygen as acceptor
    1.3.7 With an iron-sulphur protein as acceptor
    1.3.9 With other acceptors
1.4 Acting on the $CH-NH_2$ group of donors
    1.4.1 With NAD^+ or $NADP^+$ as acceptor
    1.4.2 With a cytochrome as acceptor
    1.4.3 With oxygen as acceptor

	1.4.4	With a disulphide compound as acceptor
	1.4.7	With an iron-sulphur protein as acceptor
	1.4.9	With other acceptors
1.5	Acting on the CH-NH group of donors
	1.5.1	With NAD $^+$ or NADP $^+$ as acceptor
	1.5.3	With oxygen as acceptor
	1.5.9	With other acceptors
1.6	Acting on NADH or NADPH
	1.6.1	With NAD $^+$ or NADP $^+$ as acceptor
	1.6.2	With a cytochrome as acceptor
	1.6.4	With a disulphide compound as acceptor
	1.6.5	With a quinone or related compound as acceptor
	1.6.6	With nitrogenous group as acceptor
	1.6.7	With an iron-sulphur protein as acceptor
	1.6.9	With other acceptors
1.7	Acting on other nitrogenous compounds as donors
	1.7.2	With a cytochrome as acceptor
	1.7.3	With oxygen as acceptor
	1.7.7	With an iron-sulphur protein as acceptor
	1.7.9	With other acceptors
1.8	Acting on a sulphur group of donors
	1.8.1	With NAD $^+$ or NADP $^+$ as acceptor
	1.8.2	With a cytochrome as acceptor
	1.8.3	With oxygen as acceptor
	1.8.4	With a disulphide compound as acceptor
	1.8.5	With a quinone or related compound as acceptor
	1.8.7	With an iron-sulphur protein as acceptor
	1.8.9	With other acceptors
1.9	Acting on a haem group of donors
	1.9.3	With oxygen as acceptors
	1.9.6	With a nitrogenous group as acceptor
	1.9.9	With other acceptors
1.10	Acting on diphenols and related substances as donors=
	1.10.1	With NAD$^+$ or NADP $^+$ as acceptor
	1.10.2	With a cytochrome as acceptor
	1.10.3	With oxygen as acceptor
1.11	Acting on hydrogen peroxide as acceptor

- 1.12 Acting on hydrogen as donor
  - 1.12.1 With NAD^+ or $NADP^+$ as acceptor
  - 1.12.2 With a cytochrome as acceptor
  - 1.12.7 With an iron-sulphur protein as acceptor
- 1.13 Acting on single donors with incorporation of molecular oxygen (oxygenases)
  - 1.13.11 With incorporation of two atoms of oxygen
  - 1.13.12 With incorporation of one atom of oxygen (internal monooxygenases or internal mixed function oxidases)
  - 1.13.99 Miscellaneous (requires further characterisation)
- 1.14 Acting on paired donors with incorporation of molecular oxygen
  - 1.14.11 With 2-oxoglutarate as one donor, and incorporation of one atom each of oxygen into both donors
  - 1.14.12 With NADH or NADPH as one donor, and incorporation of two atoms of oxygen into one donor
  - 1.14.13 With NADH or NADPH as one donor, and incorporation of one atom of oxygen
  - 1.14.14 With reduced flavin or flavo-protein as one donor, and incorporation of one atom of oxygen
  - 1.14.15 With a reduced iron-sulphur protein as one donor, and incorporation of one atom of oxygen
  - 1.14.16 With reduced pteridine as one donor, and incorporation of one atom of oxygen
  - 1.14.17 With ascorbate as one donor, and incorporation of one atom of oxygen
  - 1.14.18 With another compound as one donor, and incorporation of one atom of oxygen
  - 1.14.19 Miscellaneous (requires further characterization)
- 1.15 Acting on superoxide radicals as acceptor
- 1.16 Oxidizing metal ions
  - 1.16.3 With oxygen as acceptor
- 1.17 Acting on $-CH_2$ groups
  - 1.17.1 With NAD^+ or $NADP^+$ as acceptor
  - 1.17.4 With a disulphide compound as acceptor
- 1.97 Other oxidoreductases

2. TRANSFERASES

2.1 Transferring one-carbon groups
    2.1.1 Methyltransferases
    2.1.2 Hydroxymethyl-, formyl- and related transferases
    2.1.3 Carboxyl- and carbamoyltransferases
    2.1.4 Amidinotransferases
2.2 Transferring aldehyde or ketonic residues
2.3 Acyltransferases
    2.3.1 Acyltransferases
    2.3.2 Aminoacyltransferases
2.4 Glycosyltransferases
    2.4.1 Hexosyltransferases
    2.4.2 Pentosyltransferases
    2.4.3 Transfering other glycosyl groups
2.5 Transferring alkyl or aryl groups, other than methyl groups
2.6 Transferring nitrogenous groups
    2.6.1 Aminotransferases
    2.6.3 Oximinotransferases
2.7 Transferring phosphorus-containing groups
    2.7.1 Phosphotransferases with an alcohol group as acceptor
    2.7.2 Phosphotransferases with a carboxyl group as acceptor
    2.7.3 Phosphotransferases with a nitrogenous group as acceptor
    2.7.4 Phosphotransferases with a phosphate group as acceptor
    2.7.5 Phosphotransferases with regeneration of donors (apparently catalysing intramolecular transfers
    2.7.6 Diphosphotransferases
    2.7.7 Nucleotidyltransferases
    2.7.8 Transferases for other substituted phosphate groups
    2.7.9 Phosphotransferases with paired acceptors
2.8 Transferring sulphur-containing groups
    2.8.1 Sulphurtransferases
    2.8.1 Sulphotransferases
    2.8.3 CoA-transferases

3. HYDROLASES

3.1 Acting on ester bonds
    3.1.1 Carboxylic ester hydrolases
    3.1.2 Thiolester hydrolases
    3.1.3 Phosphoric monoester hydrolases
    3.1.4 Phosphoric diester hydrolases
    3.1.5 Triphosphoric monester hydrolases
    3.1.6 Sulphuric ester hydrolases
    3.1.7 Diphosphoric monoester hydrolases
    3.1.11 Exodeoxyribonucleases producing 5'-phospho-monoesters
    3.1.13 Exoribonucleases producing 5'-phosphomonoesters
    3.1.14 Exoribonucleases producing other than 5'- phosphomonoesters
    3.1.15 Exonucleases active with either ribo- or deoxyribonucleic acids and producing 5'-phosphomonoesters
    3.1.16 Exonucleases active with either ribo- or deoxyribonucleic acids and producing other than 5'-phosphomonoesters
    3.1.21 Endodeoxyribonucleases producing 5'-phosphomonoesters
    3.1.22 Endodeoxyribonucleases producing other than 5'-phosphomonoesters
    3.1.23 Site-specific endodeoxyribonuclease: cleavage is sequence-specific
    3.1.24 Site-specific endodeoxyribonuclease: cleavage is not sequence- specific
    3.1.25 Site-specific endodeoxyribonucleases: specific for altered bases
    3.1.26 Endoribonucleases producing 5'-phosphomonoesters
    3.1.27 Endoribonucleases producing other than 5'-phosphomonoesters

- 3.1.30 Endonucleases active with either ribo- or deoxyribonucleic acids and producing 5'-phosphomonoesters
- 3.1.31 Endonucleases active with either ribo- or deoxyribonucleic acids and producing other than 5'-phosphomonoesters

3.2 Acting on glycosyl compounds
- 3.2.1 Hydrolysing O-glycosyl compounds
- 3.2.2 Hydrolysing N-glycosyl compounds
- 3.2.3 Hydrolysing S-glycosyl compounds

3.3 Acting on other hands
- 3.3.1 Thioether hydrolases
- 3.3.2 Ether hydrolases

3.4 Acting on peptide bonds (peptide hydrolases)
- 3.4.11 α-Aminoacylpeptide hydrolases
- 3.4.12 Peptidylamino-acid or acylamino-acid hydrolases
- 3.4.13 Dipeptide hydrolases
- 3.4.14 Dipeptidylpeptide hydrolases
- 3.4.15 Peptidyldipeptide hydrolases
- 3.4.16 Serine carboxypeptidases
- 3.4.17 Metallo-carboxypeptidases
- 3.4.21 Serine proteinases
- 3.4.22 Thiol proteinases
- 3.4.23 Carboxyl (acid) proteinases
- 3.4.24 Metalloproteinases
- 3.4.99 Proteinases of unknown catalytic mechanism

3.5 Acting on carbon-nitrogen bonds, other than peptide bonds
- 3.5.1 In linear amides
- 3.5.2 In cyclic amides
- 3.5.3 In linear amidines
- 3.5.4 In cyclic amidines
- 3.5.5 In nitriles
- 3.5.99 In other compounds

3.6 Acting on acid anhydrides
- 3.6.1 In phosphoryl-containing anhydrides
- 3.6.2 In sulphonyl-containing anhydrides

3.7   Acting on carbon-carbon bonds
      3.7.1   In ketonic substances
3.8   Acting on halide bonds
      3.8.1   In C-halide compounds
      3.8.2   In P-halide compounds
3.9   Acting on phosphorus-nitrogen bonds
3.10 Acting on sulphur-nitrogen bonds
3.11 Acting on carbon-phosphorus bonds

4. LYASES

4.1   Carbon-carbon lyases
      4.1.1   Carboxy-lases
      4.1.2   Aldehyde-lyases
      4.1.3   Oxo-acid-lyases
      4.1.99 Other carbon-carbon lyases
4.2   Carbon-oxygen lyases
      4.2.1   Hydro-lyases
      4.2.2   Acting on polysaccharides
      4.2.99 Other carbon-oxygen lyases
4.3   Carbon-nitrogen lyases
      4.3.1   Ammonia-lyases
      4.3.2   Amidine-lyases
4.4   Carbon-Sulphur lyases
4.5   Carbon-halide lyases
4.6   Phosphorus-oxygen lyases
4.99 Other lyases

5. ISOMERASES

5.1   Racemases and epimerases
      5.1.1   Acting on amino acids and derivatives
      5.1.2   Acting on hydroxy acids and derivatives
      5.1.3   Acting on carbohydrates and derivatives
      5.1.99 Acting on other compounds
5.2   Cis-trans isomerases
5.3   Intramolecular oxidoreductases

- 5.3.1 Interconverting aldoses and ketoses
- 5.3.2 Interconverting keto- and enol-groups
- 5.3.3 Transposing C = C bonds
- 5.3.4 Transposing S = S bonds
- 5.3.99 Other intramolecular oxidoreductases

5.4 Intramolecular transferases
- 5.4.1 Transfering acyl groups
- 5.4.2 Transfering phosphoryl groups
- 5.4.3 Transfering amino groups
- 5.4.99 Transfering other groups

5.5 Intramolecular lyases

5.99 Other isomerases

6. LIGASES (SYNTHETASES)

6.1 Forming carbon-oxygen bonds
- 6.1.1 Ligases forming aminacyl-rRNA and related compounds

6.2 Forming carbon-sulphur bonds
- 6.2.1 Acid-thiol ligases

6.3 Forming carbon-nitrogen bonds
- 6.3.1 Acid-ammonia (or amine) ligases (amide synthetases)
- 6.3.2 Acid-aminoacid ligases (peptide synthetases)
- 6.3.3 Cyclo-ligases
- 6.3.4 Other carbon-nitrogen ligases
- 6.3.5 Carbon-nitrogen ligases with glutamine as amino-N-donor

6.4 Forming carbon-carbon bonds

6.5 Forming phosphate ester bonds.

II. GLOSSARY OF TERMS

Coenzyme Heat-stable, low molecular weight organic compound, required for the activity of enzymes. It is also referred to as a substance which is regenerated by other enzyme reactions in a pathway to complete a cycle and permit the repeated use of the same substrate molecule

Cofactor An inorganic essential component of an enzymatic reaction, which is not converted stoichiometrically to other forms.

Isoenzyme A physically distinct and separable form of a given enzyme present in different cell types or sub-cellular compartments of a human being. Also, it is defined to possess the ability to catalyze the enzyme characteristic reaction but differ in structure because they are encoded by distinct structural gene.

Prosthetic Group It is a tightly bound molecular structure, not part of the amino acid sequence of a protein, which is required to fulfill the catalytic function of the enzyme.

Reactant This refers to a substance, which is also synonymous with a substrate involving either direction of the enzyme action.

Substrate This refers to any molecule converted stoichiometrically to another molecule of different properties.

Ribozymes	These are ribonucleic acids (RNA's) which are not proteins but exhibit highly substrate – specific catalytic activity. They act on substrates which are limited to phosphodiester bonds of RNA's.
Competitive Inhibition	This is a type of inhibition in which the inhibitor competes with the substrate for the same binding site on the enzyme.
Uncompetitive Inhibition	A type of inhibition in which the inhibitor binds to a site other than the substrate –binding site on the enzyme-substrate complex
Non-competitive Inhibition	A type of inhibition in which the inhibitor binds to a site other than the substrate – binding site on the enzyme and enzyme-substrate complex.
Allosteric Inhibition	A type of inhibition which is exhibited by an allosteric enzyme and it is an example of a negative heterotropic cooperativity.
Allosteric Activation	This is an example of a positive heterotropic cooperativity, which is exhibited by an allosteric enzyme.
Michaelis Constant, (K_m)	This refers to the dissociation constant for the enzyme substrate complex. Quantitatively, it is the substrate concentration at which the initial velocity is half-maximal. It is a measure of affinity of an enzyme for its substrate.
Hill's Coefficient	This is an empirical parameter whose value depends on the number of substrate binding sites in an oligomeric enzyme protein, and the number and type of interactions between these binding sites.

Sequential Mechanism	A type of mechanism in bi-substrate (multisubstrate) enzyme-catalyzed reaction in which all the substrates bind to the enzyme before the first product is formed.
Ping-Pong Mechanism	A type of mechanism in multi-substrate (bi-substrate enzyme catalyzed reactions in which one or more products are released before all the substrates are added.
Allosteric Interaction	These refer to interactions between ligands bound to the protein at some distance from one another.
Homotropic Cooperativity	These are allosteric interaction between **'like'** molecules
Heterotropic Cooperativity	These are allosteric interactions between **'unlike'** molecules
Positive Cooperativity	A phenomenon exhibited by allosteric enzyme in which binding of the substrate becomes easier as the enzyme becomes more and more saturated. This occurs when the binding of one molecule of a substrate of ligand increases the affinity of the protein for other molecules of the same or different substrate or ligand.
Negative Cooperativity	A phenomenon exhibited by an allosteric enzyme in which the binding of the substrate get progressively more difficult as the enzyme becomes saturated. This occurs when the binding of one molecule of a substrate of ligand decreases the affinity of the protein for other molecules of the same or different substrate or ligand.
Cooperativity	This refers to the interaction between the binding sites present on a protein during the binding process.

INDEX

Acid-base catalysis, 115
Acid-base properties of amino acids, 27
Affinity labels, 130
Allosteric, 84
    Features of allostery, 84
    Comparison of allosteric enzymes activity, 84
Amino acid and protein metabolism, 17
Amino Acids with Negatively Charged "R Group", 24
Amino acids with Non-Polar or Hydrophobic R Groups, 23
Amino Acids with Polar but Uncharged R. Group, 23
Applications for immobilized enzymes, 161
Aromatic amino acids, 26
Assay techniques for enzyme activity, 45
Automatic titration methods, 46
Bone disease, 150
Briggs-Haldane Hypothesis, 67
Carbohydrate metabolism, 17
Cases where intermediates occurring after (ES), 69
Cellular enzymes, 146
Characterization of enzyme preparation, 21
Charge-relay system for chymotrypsin, 121
Chymotrypsin, 120

Classification and Structures of amino acids, 22
Classification of enzymes, 5
    Oxido-reductases, 5
Clinical significance of enzyme analysis, 148
Coenzymes, 33
Covalent modification, 137
Cross-Linking reagents, 131
D-amino acids, 4
Decomposing ferments, 2
Definitions of enzyme activity parameters, 42
Derivation of Michaelis-Menten Equation, 61
Derivation of rate equation for two-substrate reaction, 80
Determination of inhibitor constants, 105
Determination of the kinetic constants, 64
Distribution of enzymes, 11
Effect of pH on enzyme activity, 48
Energy-Link control, 137
Enzyme Assemblages, 32
    Multienzyme complexes, 32
    Multifunctional Enzymes, 33
Enzyme inhibition, 92
    Mixed inhibition, 104;
    Non-competitive inhibition, 97
    Types of reversible inhibition, 94

Enzyme mechanisms, 119
Enzymes bioinformatics, 161
Enzymes bound in chromatin, 13
Enzymes bound to membranes, 13
Enzymes concentrated in the
    nucleolus, 13
Enzymes in blood plasma, 145
Enzymes present in lysosomes, 15
    Hydrolysis of enzymes, 15
    Hydrolysis of glycosides, 15
    Hydrolysis of Lipids, 15
    Others, 15
Extraction of enzymes, 18
Factors affecting enzyme activity, 47
First order reaction, 57
Fractionation of enzyme preparation, 18
Gastrointestinal disease, 150
General properties of enzymes, 3
General rate equations for first order
    reactions, 59
General rate equation for second order
    reactions, 60
Genetic control and direct control of
    catalysis, 133
Groups of Enzyme Proteins, 32
    Monomeric Enzyme, 32
    Multienzyme Complexes, 32
    Oligomeric Enzymes, 32
Hanes - Woolf Plot, 65
Hemoglobin (Tetrameric Protein), 87
History of enzymology, 1
    Historical development, 1
Hormone control, 137
Hydrolases, 7
Hyperbolic competitive inhibition, 107
Identification of amino acids at the
    active site of enzymes, 126
Imino acid, 26
Immobilized enzymes, 158
Industrial uses of enzymes, 153
Inner membrane, 14

Intermembrane space, 14
Isomerases, 9
Kinetic of Bisubstrate reactions, 79
Kinetics of Ligand-binding to an
    allosteric enzyme molecule, 89
Kinetics of ligand-binding to
    hemoproteins, 86
Koshland, Nemethy and Filmer Model
    (KNF), 139
Ligand-binding to allosteric protein, 85
Ligases (Synthetases), 9
Lineweaver-Burke (Double-reciprocal
    plot) Plot, 64
Lipid metabolism, 17
Liver disease, 150
Lyases, 8
Lysozyme, 123
Marker enzyme, 12
Matrix, 14
Measurement of catalytic activity, 42
Measurement of enzyme levels, 40
    Units of measurement, 40
Measurement of rate constants, 72
Medicinal application of enzymes, 155
Metal-ion catalysis, 119
Metallo enzymes, 38
    Catalytic function, 38
    Physiological roles, 39
Molecular mechanisms of allosteric
    control, 138
Multisubstrate enzyme catalyzed
    reactions, 77
Myocardial infarction, 151
Non-linear kinetics, 81
Non-sequential mechanism, (ping-
    pong), 79
Nucleophilic and electrophonic
    catalysis (Covalent catalysis), 117
Nucleic acid synthesis, 17
Outer membrane, 15
Parabolic competitive inhibition, 107

Physiological roles of enzyme assemblages, 33
Plasma specific enzymes, 145
Polymerization - Depolymerization, 137
Preparation of immobilized enzymes, 160
Principal enzymes of the endoplasmic reticulum, 16
Prostatic disease, 151
Pseudo-substrate labels, 128
Purification of enzyme preparation, 20
    Criteria for purity, 21
Purification of enzymes, 2
Quantitative analysis of cooperativity, 88
Quantitative treatment on effect of pH on Enzyme activity, 50
Radiometry, 47
Rapid-mixing and quenching techniques, 73
    Continuous flow method, 74
    Stopped flow method, 74
    Quenching techniques, 75
Relaxation methods, 75
Reversible reaction, 70
Second order reaction, 58
Secreted enzymes, 146
Sequential mechanism, 77
    Ordered sequential, 78
    Random sequential, 78

Six major classes of enzymes, 10
Spectrofluorometry, 46
Stability of carrier-Enzyme complex, 160
Steady state kinetics for multisubstrate reactions, 82
Steady State Kinetics, 67
Structural organization of enzymes, 28
    Primary structure, 28
    Secondary structure, 28
    Quaternary structure, 30
    Tertiary structure, 30
Structure of enzymes, 22
Substrate - binding site of chymotrypsin, 121
Substrate-induced synthesis of catabolic enzymes, 134
Transferases, 6
Types of regulatory mechanism, 134
    Concerted Feedback control 136
    Cumulative Feedback control, 136
    Feedback inhibition, 134
    Sequential feedback control, 135
    Uncompetitive inhibition, 101
Urinary excretion of enzymes, 148
X-Ray crystallography of enzyme molecule, 30
Zero-order reaction, 57

www.ingramcontent.com/pod-product-compliance
Lightning Source LLC
Chambersburg PA
CBHW030925180526
45163CB00002B/467